Concordance

Concordance

A partnership in medicine-taking

Edited by

Christine Bond

BPharm, MEd, PhD, MRPharmS

Professor of Primary Care (Pharmacy)
Department of General Practice and Primary Care
School of Medicine
University of Aberdeen
Aberdeen
UK

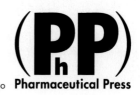

London • Chicago   **Pharmaceutical Press**

Published by the Pharmaceutical Press
Publications division of the Royal Pharmaceutical Society of Great Britain

1 Lambeth High Street, London SE1 7JN, UK
100 South Atkinson Road, Suite 206, Grayslake, IL 60030-7820, USA

© Pharmaceutical Press 2004

(**P.P**) is a trade mark of Pharmaceutical Press

First published 2004

Text design by Barker/Hilsdon, Lyme Regis, Dorset
Typeset by Photoprint, Torquay, Devon
Printed in Great Britain by TJ International, Padstow, Cornwall

ISBN 0 85369 572 5

A catalogue record for this book is available from the British Library

To all those committed to improving patient care

Contents

x Contents

Preface

In 1995 I attended a small meeting in Edinburgh, chaired by Marshall Marinker. A group of people with an interest in the effective use of medicines came together to discuss the reasons why patients do not take their medicines as directed by the prescriber. This was perceived to result in ineffective dosages, and drug wastage. In fact these discussions were the first steps on what became the concordance journey. The rest, as they say, is history and concordance is now firmly established in most healthcare professionals' vocabulary, if not understanding.

As our discussions developed, and we realised the varied and informed portfolio of research which had already been conducted in the field, the patient agenda in medicine-taking emerged as the central tenet. The publication of the *From Compliance to Concordance* report (Royal Pharmaceutical Society of Great Britain, 1997) was but one milestone on the journey, which is now being progressed by the Medicines Partnership. This current volume is a line in the sand, which recognises the dynamic nature of healthcare and concepts. By the time of publication we will almost certainly be approaching the next milestone.

Concordance is a concept which, as described by Joanne Shaw in Chapter 8, can be used with respect to both the process and the outcome of a discussion or consultation between a patient and healthcare professional. As the recent special issue of the *Pharmaceutical Journal* (October 2003) made clear, there are also many interpretations of the concordance concept *per se*, some of which adhere closely to the original underpinning beliefs, and some of which focus more on one or other aspects of the process, such as compliance with medicine-taking.

What is fundamental is that, under the direction of Marshall Marinker, a new way of looking at medicine-taking was articulated which promoted the patient's beliefs and rights, and gave them equal weight to those of the healthcare professional. As concordance evolves and blends with other paradigms in healthcare it seemed appropriate to capture, nearly 10 years on, what has been achieved. The contributors to this volume are all experts in their fields, busy people to whom I am extremely grateful for their input. Between them they reflect on what concordance means to the patient and the healthcare professional, how we operationalise it, teach it, and research it. Apart from Chapter 8, which looks at the policy issues, their individual essays are grounded in research evidence. Inevitably therefore there are some issues which we might wish to explore but which are currently unanswered.

In Chapter 1 Marshall Marinker describes in more detail than I have outlined above the genesis of concordance and his personal contribution to this. He usefully highlights the ongoing and complex relationship between compliance and concordance and helps the reader understand the confusion which still arises between these two terms, which are not, as many still believe, synonyms. In the chapter he alludes to the body of knowledge from medical sociology and health psychology, which are all antecedents of concordance and the concordance paradigm. He concludes by reminding us all of our duty to 'achieve for each patient an optimum balance between the best that medical science can offer and the health-enhancing benefits of personal enablement'.

In Chapter 2 Nicky Britten and Marjorie Weiss, in answering the question 'What is concordance?', provide some useful summaries of earlier models applied to the patient–healthcare encounter. They then review the recent research to consider the extent to which concordance is actually practised and the benefits that this might bring. Inevitably, much of this literature is medically dominated, but as professional roles change and other disciplines became more involved in front-line diagnosis and decision-making, we have to assume that at least the broad principles of their findings are transferable to other healthcare professionals such as the nurse or pharmacist. Finally in this chapter some of the continuing challenges are summarised together with solutions.

In Chapter 3 Fiona Stevenson looks at concordance from the patient's perspective. This chapter builds on Chapter 2, emphasising the different beliefs which patients, in contrast to professionals, have about medicines (also covered in Chapter 7) and their independent actions outside the consultation. There is also a reminder of the techniques they use within the consultation in order to become more involved. The wider context is also considered, with reference to recent high-profile cases which have challenged the position of trust that doctors hold in society. Also discussed are the blurring of professional boundaries, which have led to professionals other than physicians being in a position to decide about treatment, and the greater involvement of patients, reflecting a more consumerist society. As in Chapter 2, some of the barriers and challenges are reviewed from a patient's perspective and the author concludes that for concordance to succeed it requires the commitment of both patients and professionals.

The professional's perspective is addressed in detail in Chapter 4. Jon Dowell describes how the concordance paradigm is changing the behaviour of clinicians, a term which embraces both the traditional medical prescribers and the 'new' prescribers. None the less, inevitably much of the research he cites is, as in Chapter 2, based on medical interactions with patients because until recently that has been the dominant model of practice. Some of the research presented in this chapter balances the patient-centred studies reported in Chapter 3, demonstrating the range of perspectives and models which exist, and illustrating that all approaches have their strengths and weaknesses. As in the previous chapters, Jon Dowell again reiterates the barriers and challenges of concordance, this time from the prescriber's perspective, but resonating well with the issues identified by the previous authors. He concludes with useful suggestions, prescriber-led, to take concordance forward, such as patient selection, multidisciplinary working and shared record-keeping.

In Chapter 5 Alison Blenkinsopp moves the reader on from the original decision to the ongoing treatment phase. Much of this chapter is directed at opportunities for pharmacists to support that original decision, because of their role as dispensers of both the initial and future supplies of the medicine. This emphasis on the pharmacy profession also reflects the available research evidence. None the less we should bear in mind that all those involved in patient care should heed the messages in this chapter, be they doctors, nurses, pharmacists, allied health professionals or other carers. The chapter is usefully structured into sections which are based on the stages of ongoing treatment from collection of the first supply to monitoring continued treatment, and suggestions for support. At all these stages healthcare professionals have a role to listen and respond to patient beliefs and facilitate greater concordance in medicine-taking.

In Chapter 6 Marjorie Weiss addresses the important questions of how we can help health professionals to learn about concordance. The text draws on the medical, nursing and pharmacy literature and includes practical advice and role-play examples. Whilst the chapter does not avoid the potential problems surrounding the teaching of an abstract and still evolving concept such as concordance, it also manages to make these potential weaknesses a strength in increasing understanding of the topic. It also usefully integrates its approach with other recent advances in the teaching of communication skills, including structured frameworks on which to base the consultation and an awareness of the effect of personal beliefs. It has the current learner-centred approach to education and a useful analogy is drawn between this and concordance itself. Once again the nebulous nature of concordance poses new challenges for assessment, and examples of how this might be achieved are integrated with current educational approaches.

In Chapter 7 Robert Horne and John Weinman take a classical approach to research by first identifying the research questions we might ask about concordance. In articulating these questions, as any researcher knows, it is necessary to unpick the process under study so that we can identify measurable units. The first half of this chapter does this with particular reference to what the authors define as informed adherence. They make it clear that, whilst informed adherence is not concordance *per se*, it is one component of concordance and its measurement will contribute to a research agenda. Other components of the concordance model ultimately have to be similarly analysed and techniques developed to measure the individual units. Some aspects of adherence have already been explored using psychological models and the authors lead us through these to help us operationalise the elements of the consultation to be measured. In this regard this chapter complements the overview of the patient's perspective in Chapter 3 and the prescriber's perspective in Chapter 4. This theoretical approach is consistent with recent Medical Research Council guidance on evaluating complex interventions. In the concluding section the authors present a schema for research to address the input, the process and the outcomes of the consultation, with respect to concordance. They again challenge the belief that concordance is always the best solution for both patient and population. This may appear to run counter to the concordance ideal, but it is about recognising and being alert to both positive and negative outcomes.

In the final chapter Joanne Shaw, Director of the Medicines Partnership, summarises the current policy framework, which is taking concordance forward. She ties the development of the concordance paradigm into two other cultural developments relating to patient and public involvement and patient safety. She reminds us of the huge mountain to climb to embed concordance into practice and the long-term nature of the enterprise which will depend largely on the education of patients and professionals. She also emphasises the need to have a multiplicity of approaches to effect change, and reminds us of the need to ensure that policy, communication and research, and models of good practice are all essential components of change. This chapter differs from most of the others. It is about what is happening now. It is not based on research evidence but is a description of how research can lead to new behavioural beliefs which then need to be translated into practice. This is a big agenda with many challenges. It is about the future and how we ensure that the ethos of concordance will be sustained whilst all around there is constant change.

Many questions still remain unanswered: these remain a challenge, but should not be seen as insurmountable barriers or reasons to abandon our ideals. One of the biggest conundrums remaining is the medicolegal position of the healthcare professional if he/she supports a patient who decides not to persist with the evidence-based route advised. Issues such as this will become clearer as both professionals and patients continue to explore and respect each other's perspectives. As professionals and academics we have a responsibility to share, publish and learn from such interactions so that our combined understanding continually improves.

I hope this volume will capture some key elements of concordance and provide the springboard for further development in effective patient care. It should be of relevance to practitioners and policy-makers, educationalists and students, and of course patients. It is time to take stock and reflect where we are, and where we want to go; the goal is better patient care.

Reference

Royal Pharmaceutical Society of Great Britain (1997). *From Compliance to Concordance: Achieving Shared Goals in Medicine Taking*. London: RPSGB.

Christine Bond
April 2004

About the editor

Christine Bond has worked for Glaxo Research Laboratories, had extensive locum community pharmacist experience, and is now Professor of Primary Care: Pharmacy, and Deputy Head of Department in the Department of General Practice and Primary Care, University of Aberdeen. She is Head of Undergraduate General Practice teaching and has an extensive research portfolio, with well over 100 publications. Her main research interests are in the optimum use of medicines, both prescribed and over-the-counter, and the contribution of community pharmacy to the wider primary healthcare agenda. She is currently seconded to Grampian Health Board as a part-time Consultant in Pharmaceutical Public Health. She was a member of the original From Compliance to Concordance Working Party. Her current national responsibilities include the Chief Scientist Office (Scottish Executive) Health Services Research Committee, the Main Research Ethics Committee for Scotland and the UK Steering Group to Review Access to Yellow Card Data. She is an elected member of the Royal Pharmaceutical Society of Great Britain Scottish Executive.

Contributors

Alison Blenkinsopp
Professor of the Practice of Pharmacy, Department of Medicines Management, Keele University, Staffs, UK

Christine Bond
Professor of Primary Care, Head of Teaching, Department of General Practice and Primary Care, University of Aberdeen, Aberdeen, UK

Nicky Britten
Professor of Applied Health Care Research, Institute of Clinical Education, Peninsula Medical School, Universities of Exeter and Plymouth, St Luke's Campus, Exeter, Devon, UK

Jon Dowell
Senior Lecturer, Tayside Centre for General Practice, University of Dundee, Dundee, UK

Robert Horne
Professor of Psychology in Health Care, Director, Centre for Health Care Research (CHCR), University of Brighton, Falmer, Brighton, UK

Marshall Marinker
Visiting Professor of General Practice, GKT, King's College, University of London, UK

Joanne Shaw
Director, Medicines Partnership, 1 Lambeth High Street, London SE1 7JN, UK

Fiona Stevenson
Lecturer in Medical Sociology, Department of Primary Care & Population Sciences, Royal Free and University College School of Medicine, UK

John Weinman
Professor of Psychology as applied to Medicine, Department of Psychology (at Guy's), Institute of Psychiatry, London, UK

Marjorie Weiss
Senior Lecturer, School of Pharmacy, University of Bath, Bath, UK

1

From compliance to concordance: a personal view

Marshall Marinker

In 1995 the Royal Pharmaceutical Society of Great Britain, in partnership with Merck Sharp & Dohme, undertook an inquiry into what was known about the difficulties patients have in taking medicines as they are prescribed. The intention was to review the extent, causes and consequences of this 'non-compliance'. On the basis of this inquiry we were to make recommendations about how to improve the taking of medicines. In the first half of 1995 a steering group was set up, and I was invited to chair it.

Instinctively I found myself somewhat reluctant to accept the invitation. This, despite my general awareness of the consequences of non-compliance – that the non-compliant patient fails to achieve the full potential of benefit from the medicines prescribed. My reservations stemmed from two pre-existing points of view. Firstly, my own professional experiences, and the ensuing body of theory in academic general practice about the nature of the clinical encounter in generalist medicine, suggested how pervasive is the uncertainty that links the patient's perception of illness, the doctor's diagnosis, the choice of treatment and the subsequent history. The goal of compliance with the prescription therefore seemed too-often rooted in rather shifting ground.

More than 30 years ago, contributing to an international conference on the exponential explosion of tranquilliser-prescribing, I suggested that the doctor's seemingly rational statement: 'I've listened to your story, Mrs Smith, and you are clearly a case of anxiety. You had better have some Librium,' concealed a more truthful exposition: 'I've listened to your story, Mrs Smith, and you are clearly a case of Librium. You had better have some anxiety.'

The act of prescribing is complex and cannot invariably be relied upon to provide a copper-bottomed standard for judging the appropriateness of medicine-taking. The range of variation in the diagnoses that doctors make, particularly in relation to the vast majority of illnesses that are not readily ascribed to well-researched physical pathologies, is very broad. In so many of these cases the diagnosis is not so much the basis for the prescription, as its alibi.

Secondly, I had long regarded non-compliance as something more than a procedural accident – the result of misunderstood instructions, or of the patient's physical, social or psychological inability to follow them. Without knowing as much as I ought to have done about how patients feel about taking medicines, I had long sensed that non-compliance was often a positive act – albeit not always consciously reasoned. All medicine-taking involves a balance of risk between the damage of the disease process, unmodified by medication, on the one hand, and the potential damage which might be inflicted by the medicine, on the other. Intentional non-compliance therefore simply represents a particular choice of risk – a defence mechanism against a perceived (and sometimes an actual) iatrogenic threat. Therefore, in our attempts to improve the quality and outcome of medicine-taking, an estimate of compliance was arguably not the only, and not always the best, yardstick. If the professionals wished to dismantle this (often unconscious) defence against the threat from medication, how confident could we be that we were offering something better?

This reluctance on my part to explore non-compliance and to seek measures to reduce its impact on treatment was to have strong resonances with everything that I subsequently learned about the scale of non-compliance, and about the many forms of resistance that people have to taking their prescribed medicines as advised.

My chairmanship of this initial 1995 steering group, and a number of subsequent committees charged with similar tasks, was to provide me with a rich education in the researches around medicine-taking carried out from many different theoretical standpoints – in pharmacy, clinical pharmacology, health economics, medical sociology and health psychology. For this education I have to thank the steering group and their contacts, the many authors of this volume, and the patients' representatives who were later to take me to task.

The steering committee began by consulting a number of healthcare professionals and researchers known to be concerned with this issue. Experts from the hospital specialties, general practice, nursing, pharmacy, health economics, social policy analysis and others met to discuss their experiences and insights. Our group was then succeeded by a working party, made up of many of the leading experts whom we had consulted. The task was to commission additional reviews of the literature, to deliberate further, and to bring out a report.

In 1997 we published a consultative document, *Partnership in Medicine Taking* (Royal Pharmaceutical Society of Great Britain, 1997a). Copies were circulated to a variety of relevant organisations and individuals. The analysis of some 90 written comments was followed by an intensive round of consultations. It was only at this late juncture, with (as we then thought) the outline of our report clearly laid out in the consultative document, that my working party arranged to spend a day with representatives of patients' groups.

The ensuing meeting was revelatory. Here at last we encountered a group of people whose suffering from severe long-term medical conditions had given them practical experiences, and a profound understanding of the problems of medicine-taking. Their insights gave sharp meaning to all that we had been learning from the researchers about the patients' beliefs, priorities, methods of reasoning and decision-taking about medicines – rationalities that were for the most part obscured behind the formalised games of the medical encounter. Much of this is now rehearsed in the following chapters of this book.

At this 1997 meeting with 'representative' patients, the conclusions of all this research were reconfirmed at first hand. We also encountered the anger and frustration of patients who had felt infantilised or ignored by health professionals whose lofty intentions were too-often unmatched by the appropriate knowledge and skills in this regard. We promised that our final report would take on board what we had learned that day. I believe that we kept our promise.

The implied aim of our consultative document had remained what it had always been in the previous research and review literature: to improve compliance. By the time we published our final report, *From Compliance to Concordance: Achieving Shared Goals in Medicine Taking*, more than the title had been changed. So had our aims. In advocating 'concordance', the report was not simply offering an alternative term, a more politically acceptable way of talking about compliance. Rather, what was now being urged was a radical change in culture – in research, in teaching and in practice. We were advocating a new balance in the relationship between prescribing and medicine-taking, between patient and prescriber.

Social scientist researchers into medicine-taking had many years ago preferred the verb 'adhere' to 'comply': we adhere to agreements; we comply with instructions. 'Adherence' allowed the social scientists to distance themselves from a doctor-centred and paternalistic view of the clinical transaction. Words matter.

It is our vocabularies that define and delimit the spaces of the imagination – no less in scientific research and professional practice than in art and philosophy. The use of the term 'adherence' was an advance, but its limitations, although not obvious, were substantial. The notion of 'adherence' still failed to encompass the possibility that taking medicines to best effect in purely biotechnical terms was not necessarily the one desired outcome.

I lighted upon the term 'medicines concordance' while drafting my preliminary notes for our report. Eureka! 'Concordance' seemed to catch what we had been talking about – the subtleties of balance between the concerns of prescriber and patient, a new resolution which went beyond bioscience, and indeed beyond the cruder expressions of so-called patient autonomy.

At our next meeting the members of our working party enthusiastically endorsed the term. And then one of our group, Sir Charles George, informed me that while he approved the term 'it was of course first used in this sense by Barbara Hulka (1976) and colleagues some twenty years ago'.

Most originality is unconscious plagiarism. Hulka *et al.* (1976), in a paper on patient–physician communication, reflected that compliance and non-compliance were both patient-related phenomena and that non-compliant behaviour represented the patient's choice. They wrote: 'Recognition of this interaction broadens the concept of patient compliance to one of physician–patient concordance.'

But in the section headed 'Discussion', the writers revealed that they were still focused on the desirability of following doctor's orders:

> Rarely have researchers and practitioners studied the extent to which apparent non-compliance is merely the lack of congruity between what the patient thinks he is supposed to do, and what the physician thinks the patient is doing. Just as it is the patient's responsibility to follow the physician's instructions, it should also be the physician's responsibility to know if and how often the patient takes his drugs. Recognition of this interaction broadens the concept of patient compliance to one of physician–patient concordance.

And they tellingly concluded: 'If instructions are to be followed, they must be understood by the patient. This may require written instructions or an additional provider to insure comprehension of the information transmitted.'

The origination of the term applied to medicine-taking then belongs to Hulka *et al*. But the definitions which we now gave in our report went far beyond what Hulka *et al*. considered. They were concerned with the provision of better communications and clearer instructions in pursuit of compliance. In *From Compliance to Concordance* (Royal Pharmaceutical Society of Great Britain, 1997b) compliance remained a desired outcome of the prescribing encounter, but it was no longer either a sufficient, nor indeed a necessary one.

We gave the following depiction of compliance:

> The patient presents with a significant medical problem for which there is a potentially helpful treatment. What the doctor or other health care professional brings to the situation – scientific evidence and technical expertise – is classed as the solution. What the patient brings – 'health beliefs' based on such qualities as culture, personality, family tradition and experience – is classed by clinicians as the impediment to the solution. The only sensible way out of this difficulty would appear to be to bring the patient's response to the doctor's diagnosis and proposed treatment as far as possible into line with what medical science suggests.

This we set against our depiction of concordance:

> The clinical encounter is concerned with two sets of contrasted but equally cogent health beliefs – that of the patient, and that of the doctor. The task of the patient is to convey her or his health beliefs to the doctor; and of the doctor, to enable this to happen. The task of the doctor or other prescriber is to convey his or her (professionally informed) health beliefs to the patient; and of the patient, to entertain these. The intention is to assist the patient to make as informed a choice as possible about the diagnosis and treatment, about benefit and risk, and to take full part in a therapeutic alliance. *Although reciprocal, this is an alliance in which the most important determinations are agreed to be those that are made by the patient.*

To make crystal clear our intent, the report went on to say that though 'concordance' was intended to convey respect for the health beliefs of both doctor and patient, it did not necessarily predicate a resolution of the differences between them on the terms of 'superior' contemporary medical evidence.

In the 6 years since our report was published there has been substantial progress. The Royal Pharmaceutical Society of Great Britain established a Concordance Co-ordinating Group. Again, I was invited to chair. Our task was to persuade government to recognise the scale and seriousness of the gap between the therapeutic potential of modern medicines and their suboptimal use by patients. We asked government to back our analysis of the problem and support our outlined programme of reform which included public awareness, professional skills, and research and development.

The then Junior Health Minister was Lord (Philip) Hunt, who had had a distinguished career in health service management. He and his ministerial colleagues accepted our arguments, earmarked funds, and then in January 2002 a Director of Medicines Partnership was appointed. Joanne Shaw came to the role with a very impressive record in change management, and a considerable understanding of the issues derived from the health-related work she had led at the Audit Commission. She and her team are advised and supported by a government Task Force co-chaired by Jim Smith, Chief Pharmaceutical Officer, Department of Health, England, and myself.

There are problems embedded in the idea of concordance which are reflected in this introductory chapter: in my initial reluctance to enquire into medicine-taking; in the confusion that arises when people employ the 'mood music' of concordance, while holding to the (understandable but misplaced) belief that the intention is simply to achieve compliance; in the meaning originally attached to the term concordance by Hulka and her associates.

As I write, Medicines Partnership has achieved much in its first 2 years. The initiative is, I believe, destined to prosper with continuing material and moral support from government and a variety of stakeholders. Many sensible reforms will be required. These include more accessible, sensitive and appropriate information for patients; the development of new consultation skills; a re-engineering of the roles and tasks of the professionals, and of services for patients.

Public policy, the evaluation of new medicines and experimental projects in the delivery of health service all need to take concordance into account. In the flurry of all these endeavours it may be hard, but it will be necessary to return time and again to a consideration of what we mean by concordance. In the laudable attempt to simplify the message, sometimes the complex meaning can become 'dumbed down' and then so easily lost. Concordance must not become compliance with a smiling face.

Also, it will be damaging prematurely to translate what is a difficult professional challenge into a prescriptive clinical guideline. Some years ago I described concordance as a good idea in the making. That is how I hope it will continue. The idea and the competencies must develop in sympathy with its essential philosophy – that of a working partnership between patients and professionals. The aim is to achieve for each patient an optimum balance between the best that medical science can offer and the health-enhancing benefits of personal enablement.

References

Hulka B, Cassel J, Kupper L, Burdett E J (1976). Communication, compliance and concordance between physicians and patients with prescribed medications. *Am J Public Health* 66: 847–853.

Royal Pharmaceutical Society of Great Britain (1997a). *Partnership in Medicine Taking*. London: RPSGB.

Royal Pharmaceutical Society of Great Britain (1997b). *From Compliance to Concordance: Achieving Shared Goals in Medicine Taking*. London: RPSGB.

2

What is concordance?

Nicky Britten and Marjorie Weiss

Introduction

The publication of the concordance report (Royal Pharmaceutical Society of Great Britain, 1997) signalled a new way of thinking about how patients and professionals communicate about medicine-taking. For some practitioners and researchers, concordance represented a challenging new idea. For others, it seemed familiar due to its similarity to other models that had been discussed in the literature for some time.

Unlike compliance, concordance has understanding, and respect, for the patient's view at its core. It involves the healthcare professional eliciting and understanding the patient's view and for these two equal partners in the interaction to agree a management plan that incorporates both their respective views. If such agreement is not possible, it is about an agreement to differ, with the onus on the healthcare professional to offer future discussions should the patient wish to revisit the issue. The model of concordance overtly recognises that the patient makes the final decision about whether or not to take medicines. It aims to make explicit any differences between patient and professional, and to promote decision-making processes that respect these differences. In the model of compliance, a patient who does not take medicine as prescribed is seen as being wilfully disobedient to the prescriber's wishes. This underlines an important distinction between compliance and concordance: concordance focuses on the consultation process while compliance refers to a specific patient behaviour.

Researchers in the field of communication have developed a number of conceptual models to describe relationships between patients and professionals. The value of these conceptual models is in being able to identify good practice when it occurs, facilitate its adoption in clinical practice, and research its impact on patient outcomes. Some models have attempted to describe the relationship in general terms, and some have concentrated on certain aspects of the consultation, such as information-giving or decision-making. Some models have been developed for the purposes of teaching (Silverman *et al.*, 1998) and not all of them have been evaluated empirically.

In this chapter, various models of the patient–practitioner relationship will be described. Their relevance for and similarity to concordance will be elucidated, and the evidence for each of them will be considered. The main difference between concordance and other models is its focus on prescribing and medicine-taking.

Concordance was introduced, and is discussed here, in terms of face-to-face consultations between individual patients and individual professionals, with a focus on the prescribing decision, but it could apply equally to other 'treatments', such as lifestyle change. Likewise, there is no reason why the concept of concordance could not be applied at a group, community or societal level when considering, for example, the question of MMR vaccination (Vernon, 2003). This wider definition is, however, beyond the scope of the present chapter.

Models of the patient–practitioner relationship

Paternalism

Paternalism is the traditional model of the doctor–patient relationship in which the doctor is the expert and the patient's role is to comply with the doctor's advice. It is within this model that the term 'patient' most accurately sits, with the implications of passivity and obedience. It is within this model that the term 'compliance' also arose, to denote the patient's obedience to the doctor's instructions. Stimson (1974), for example, criticised the image of the ideal patient in compliance research as a passive, obedient and unquestioning recipient of medical instructions. The whole point of concordance, therefore, is that it is different from the model of paternalism.

The term 'concordance' is sometimes, mistakenly, taken as a synonym for compliance (Haynes *et al.*, 2001), perhaps because it had its origins in a review of compliance. While compliance refers to something that patients do or do not do with their medicines, concordance refers to a relationship between two or more parties. A patient can be non-compliant but an individual cannot be non-concordant. Only a consultation, or a discussion, can be non-concordant. Concordance also differs from compliance in acknowledging and valuing the patient's perspective. The two terms are related, however, as concordance may well lead to improved prescribing and medicine-taking, although this has not yet been established.

This is not to say that there is no place for what Coulter (2002) refers to as professional choice.⟨In some situations, such as emergencies, or if the patient genuinely prefers it, it is appropriate for the professional to make decisions without the patient's active involvement.⟩Thus paternalism, or professional choice, is compatible with concordance provided that this reflects the patient's preference, and this preference has been elicited from the patient.

Paternalism is not only the traditional model of the doctor–patient relationship, but is also considered to be the most common one (Roter and Hall, 1992). Thus the recent review of interventions to improve adherence (Haynes *et al.*, 2001), which concluded that the full benefits of medications cannot be realised at currently achievable levels of adherence, reflects the inadequacy of the paternalistic model for ensuring best use of medicines.

Consumer choice

If the paternalistic model reflects the situation in which the professional has most control and the patient least control, the consumer choice model is at the opposite end of the continuum. In this model, the professional has a low degree of control while the patient has most control. It is part of a widespread discourse and ideology of consumerism that is by no means unique to healthcare (Fairclough, 1989). Within healthcare, the discourse of consumerism is used in relation to user involvement, the internal market and so on. However, there is little evidence that the model of consumerism is relevant in situations where people are ill or do not have genuine choices, or that it provides an accurate description of many one-to-one consultations.

Model of clinical negotiation

The model of clinical negotiation advocated by Katon and Kleinman (1981) comes close to concordance. This is an eight-stage model of the clinical encounter which begins with the physician eliciting the patient's explanatory model, after which the physician presents his or her explanatory model. This model draws on the anthropological literature about lay and professional explanatory models. Katon and Kleinman explained that the physician needs to elicit the patient's model first, to avoid contaminating or inhibiting the patient by presenting the physician's model first. Following this exchange of views, the model described the steps needed to arrive at a negotiated agreement, acknowledging the possibility that such an agreement might not be possible. However, this model was not just about prescribing or medicine-taking, but about the overall clinical encounter, of which decisions around the prescription are but one part.

Patient-centredness

Concordance also shares features with the patient-centred clinical method advocated by Stewart *et al.* (2003). The patient-centred method is concerned with much more than prescribing and medicine-taking. In a recent paper, Stewart outlines the key features of an international definition of patient-centred care in which a professional's task within the consultation has the following core elements (Stewart, 2001):

1.   Explore the patient's main reason for the visit, concerns and need for information.
2.   Seek an integrated understanding of the patient's world, that is, the whole person, emotional needs and life issues.
3.   Find common ground on what the problem is and mutually agree on management.
4.   Enhance prevention and health promotion.
5.   Enhance the continuing relationship between the patient and the doctor.

Its third element, finding common ground regarding management, requires patients and physicians to reach a mutual understanding and agreement on the nature of the problems, the goals and priorities of treatment and/or management, and their respective roles (Stewart *et al.*, 2003). This approach is more strategic or goal-oriented than the shared decision-making approach (see below) in that there is less emphasis on the specific skills needed to achieve the desired aim of patient-centredness. For example, it eschews identifying, or advocating the need for, specific skills such as bargaining or negotiating which may need to occur between doctor and patient to resolve differing goals (Stewart *et al.*, 2003: 96). Instead, the approach argues more abstractly for the participants to move towards a meeting of minds or to find common ground. A similar overarching approach is found in Mead and Bower's review of the conceptual framework for patient-centredness. They identify five conceptual dimensions (Mead and Bower, 2000):

1.   to adopt a biopsychosocial perspective
2.   to understand the individual's experience of illness or see the 'patient as person'
3.   to share power and responsibility in the encounter

4. to develop a therapeutic alliance in which the importance of the doctor and patient relationship is recognised
5. to acknowledge the 'doctor as person', in which doctor subjectivity and a greater self-awareness of the influence of the doctor's emotional responses are seen as an inherent, and potentially valuable, part of the patient-centred process

Both Stewart's and Mead and Bower's descriptions of patient-centredness resonate well with the themes of patient empowerment, therapeutic alliance and the importance of the patient perspective that form an integral part of the concordant approach. Unlike the shared decision-making models, patient-centredness places less emphasis on specific consultation skills or the need for high-quality patient information to facilitate this process.

Shared (and informed) decision-making

The model that might seem closest to concordance is shared decision-making (Charles *et al.*, 1997, 1999). Earlier versions of this model are evident in Tuckett *et al.*'s (1985) notion of meetings between experts and Roter and Hall's (1992) model of mutuality. The shared decision-making model has been specified more precisely than the previous two models and includes four necessary characteristics (Charles *et al.*, 1999):

1. At a minimum, both the physician and patient are involved in the treatment decision-making process.
2. Both the physician and patient share information with each other.
3. Both the physician and patient take steps to participate in the decision-making process by expressing treatment preferences.
4. A treatment decision is made and both the physician and patient agree on the treatment to implement.

However, it is possible to have concordance without shared decision-making, as some patients may not want to share decisions, preferring instead that the practitioner takes responsibility. The key issue is for the patient's preference for involvement in the decision-making process to be elicited, with the consultation process reflecting the patient's wishes. Therefore a consultation with a physician adopting a more paternalistic approach can still be concordant should this be the approach the patient prefers. In these situations, engagement with patients' views about medicines is still necessary to avoid misunderstandings that could lead to non-adherence (Britten *et al.*, 2000). In the context of long-term treatment of chronic problems, new decisions are not necessarily being made at each consultation. The need for mutual understanding remains, as a patient's symptoms or situation may be evolving. Although there may not be an overt discussion of treatment choices in the consultation, the patient is always making an implicit decision to take, or to continue to take, the medication.

Decision-making and the wide applicability of concordance are also pertinent to the related issue of equipoise. Equipoise is discussed in the context of the competences of shared decision-making, as described by Elwyn *et al.* (2000) (Box 2.1). (See page 96 for an explanation of the distinction between *competences* and *competencies.)*

Elwyn and Charles (2001) define clinical equipoise to occur 'when the professional admits that there are two or more possible directions and that the clinician does not have a strong view towards any given option'. Concordance, in contrast, takes a broader perspective, encompassing a greater range of clinical conditions than those with true clinical equipoise. Eliciting the patient's view, and involving those patients in decision-making who would like to be involved, is also appropriate in situations where best clinical practice is known. Patients may sometimes reject what may be considered the best clinical option even when they fully understand the nature and consequences of this decision. Equally, concordance does not detract from the autonomy of the doctor who may wish to document such events fully or refuse to prescribe in situations considered to be medically unsafe. This can concern some healthcare professionals who believe they may be at risk of litigation should a

---

Box 2.1 Stages and competences of involving patients in healthcare decisions

1. Implicit or explicit involvement of patients in decision-making process
2. Agree and define the problem that needs a decision process
3. Explore ideas, fears and expectations of the problem and possible treatments
4. Portrayal of equipoise and options
5. Identify preferred format and provide tailor-made information
6. Checking process: understanding of information and reactions (e.g. ideas, fears and expectations of possible options)
7. Checking process: acceptance of process and decision-making role preference, involving patients to the extent they desire to be involved
8. Make, discuss or defer decisions
9. Arrange follow-up

Reproduced with permission from Elwyn *et al.* (2000).

patient who has refused best medical treatment suffer an adverse event as a result. However, as discussed later in this chapter, research evidence suggests that good communication consultation skills militate against the likelihood of such malpractice claims (Levinson *et al.*, 1997). In this context, concordance is about raising to a level of explicitness those decision-making processes, by both the patient and healthcare professional, which were previously unelaborated or occurred outwith the consultation.

Elwyn and Edwards drew upon the work of Towle and Godolphin (1999) for the development of their competences. Towle and Godolphin describe this framework of informed shared decision-making as 'a coherent process and an accomplishment of any doctor–patient encounter in which a substantive decision is made about treatment or investigation for which reasonable choices exist' (Box 2.2).

Box 2.2   Competencies for physicians for informed shared decision-making

1.   Develop a partnership with the patient
2.   Establish or review the patient's preferences for information (such as amount or format)
3.   Establish or review the patient's preferences for role in decision-making (such as risk-taking and degree of involvement of self and others) and the existence and nature of any uncertainty about the course of action to take
4.   Ascertain and respond to patient's ideas, concerns and expectations (such as about disease management options)
5.   Identify choices (including ideas and information that the patient may have) and evaluate the research evidence in relation to the individual patient
6.   Present (or direct patient to) evidence, taking into account competencies 2 and 3 and framing effects (how presentation of the information may influence decision-making). Help patient to reflect on and assess the impact of alternative decisions with regard to his or her values and lifestyle
7.   Make or negotiate a decision in partnership with the patient and resolve conflict
8.   Agree an action plan and complete arrangements for follow-up

Informed shared decision-making may also:

- involve a team of health professionals
- involve others (partners, family)
- differ across cultural, social and age groups

Reproduced with permission from Towle and Godolphin (1999).

Partnership, an informed patient and explicitness of discussion regarding information needs and preferences, are prominent themes of this model which have relevance for concordance. Based upon their own interview work, Elwyn and Charles (2001) revised this framework to outline the series of competences shown in Box 2.1. More recently this approach has become aligned with the theory of 'evidence-based patient choice', which brings together the concepts of evidence-based medicine and patient-centred care. As discussed by Ford *et al.* (2002), in the medical consultation, evidence-based patient choice means providing patients with evidence-based information in a way that facilitates their ability to make choices or decisions about their healthcare. In common with concordance, this approach emphasises respect for patient autonomy. As explained by Ford, 'patients should be in a position to choose whether to accept an intervention or not as part of their general right to determine their own lives' (Ford *et al.*, 2002). Implicit within this model is a recognition that individuals differ both in what they value and in their willingness to take risks (Hope, 1996).

The literature on shared decision-making and evidence-based patient choice does however focus on the role of the professional rather more than on the role of the patient and to this extent they are doctor-centred instruments (Britten, 2003). Towle and Godolphin (1999) have recognised this and developed a preliminary list of seven competencies which will be necessary for patients to engage in informed shared decision-making:

1.   Define (for oneself) the preferred doctor–patient relationship.
2.   Find a physician and establish, develop and adapt a partnership.
3.   Articulate (for oneself) health problems, feelings, beliefs and expectations in an objective and systematic manner.
4.   Communicate with the physician in order to understand and share relevant information clearly and at the appropriate time in the medical interview.
5.   Access information.
6.   Evaluate information.
7.   Negotiate decisions, give feedback, resolve conflict and agree on an action plan (Towle and Godolphin, 1999).

More accessible patient information may be the best way forward to facilitate greater patient involvement and improve a patient's competence in a shared decision-making approach. Holmes-Rovner *et al.* (2001) have suggested a basic template for patient-oriented evidence, readily accessible by the public and added to systematic reviews and other key assessments of health technology. These summaries of clinical effectiveness will offer patients information about treatment alternatives, the benefits and harms of each, and information enabling them to clarify personal values regarding different outcomes (Holmes-Rovner *et al.,* 2001).

To what extent is concordance being practised?

A comprehensive study of British general practice carried out by Tuckett and colleagues (1985) showed that most consultations could not be characterised as a meeting between experts. The authors concluded that doctors and patients did not share or exchange ideas to a very great degree, and that the few attempts made to establish the patient's ideas and explanations were brief to the point of being absent. Fifteen years later, a study specifically concerned with doctor–patient communication about drugs in British general practice showed that the lack of discussion of patients' ideas about medicines led to misunderstandings and thence to potential or actual non-adherence (Britten *et al.,* 2000). A range of misunderstandings was identified, all of which could be characterised by a lack of patient participation in the consultation, and all of which were associated with subsequent problems with medicine-taking (Box 2.3).

The same study showed that these consultations could not be described as demonstrating shared decision-making, because the doctors and patients did not exchange views to any great extent (Stevenson *et al.,* 2000). In an earlier work, Makoul *et al.* (1995) explored the communication about medicines using videotapes of 271 doctor–patient consultations. The patient's ability to follow the treatment plan was discussed in only 8% of the recorded consultations. They also found that doctors consistently overestimated the extent to which they engaged in important communication tasks. For example, although doctors thought they had found out what the patient thought about the medication in 49% of the consultations, from the video data this was evident in only 34%.

Other work, focused less specifically on medicine-taking, supports this view. Braddock, using his informed decision-making model, found that of the 1057 audiotaped doctor–patient encounters recorded, covering 3552 clinical decisions, only 9% met the authors' definition of completeness for informed decision-making (Braddock *et al.,* 1999). An exploration of the patient's preferred role in decision-making occurred in 5.9% of these consultations. In a recent review of the patient-

---

Box 2.3   An example of misunderstanding in the consultation

Patient 40
Mrs X is a 67-year-old retired cleaner. She has had rheumatoid arthritis for 7 months and has difficulty walking and getting about. She takes a range of drugs, including painkillers, and has gold injections at the hospital. She is also worried that she is losing her hair.

Doctor 14
Dr A is a female doctor in a single-handed rural practice.

Summary of misunderstanding
The patient is uncertain about the cause of her hair loss. In the consultation she asks whether the hair loss is due to the drugs, and the doctor replies with a question about steroid injections. In the postconsultation interview the patient attributes the hair loss to her gold injections and decides to discontinue them.

Consultation
Patient: And there's another thing. I'm losing my hair. Erm, is it the medication or is it, erm, the arthritis or what? Could it be? I don't know … Mm. I mean I know I've never had a good head of hair but …
Doctor: You've just had steroid injections, haven't you? You haven't been taking steroids by mouth, have you?
Patient: No.
Doctor: No, I doubt if it's the injections. Er … how many have you had?
Patient: Erm. I've had … I've had four, I think.
Doctor: Four altogether?
Patient: Mm. Do you think it's them then?
Doctor: It's … it's possible but … erm … on the other hand, it may be again just one of those things …
Patient: Mm.
Doctor: … that people do tend to get thinner hair as they get older.

Postconsultation interview with patient
Patient: Well, I did mention about losing my hair and she thought it was the injections that I've been having. So I won't be having any more of those.
Interviewer: What were the injections? I don't think we talked about those.
Patient: Well, I used to have one every time I went to the hospital … I think they're called gold injections.
Interviewer: Is that for the arthritis?
Patient: Yes.
Interviewer: So how often have you had that before?
Patient: I've had four altogether.
Interviewer: And she thinks that's what's causing your hair to fall out?   ⇨

Box 2.3 (cont.)

Patient: She thinks that's what it is. She's not sure, but that's what she thinks.
Interviewer: Right. And were they helping at all – the injections?
Patient: Cor, they're marvellous. They last a month and you don't get any pain at all.
Interviewer: So it's a bit of a shame not to be able to have any more then?
Patient: Mmm ... I'm not having any more, I'd rather keep me hair!

Reproduced with permission from Britten *et al.* (2000).

centredness of videos submitted as part of Membership in the Royal College of General Practitioners, the authors concluded that the performance of patient-centred skills could only be demonstrated to a limited extent (Campion *et al.*, 2002). This study reported that involving patients in decision-making through the sharing of management options was not seen at all in the videos submitted by 14% of doctors, with only 36% showing this ability in three or more of the five consultations submitted. A lack of information-sharing and the tendency for doctors to pursue their own agenda was reiterated in the interesting study by Marvel *et al.* (1999) which explored the extent to which physicians solicit patients' concerns. They found that patients' initial statements of concern were completed in 28% (74/199) of the patient–physician interviews, with physicians redirecting the patient's opening statement after a mean of 23.1 seconds (Marvel *et al.*, 1999). While low, this figure is an improvement compared with the earlier 1984 study which showed that redirection by the physician occurred after a mean time of only 18 seconds (Beckman and Frankel, 1984).

Patient passivity is a widespread phenomenon (Kjellgren *et al.*, 2000). In a study of communication about antihypertensive medication in Sweden, physicians and patients were found to talk about medication very differently. Patients talked about the experiences of being on medication while physicians focused on pharmacological effect and dosage. Patients had a very fragmentary understanding of their medication and their questions mainly referred to unwanted effects (Kjellgren *et al.*, 1998). In a series of papers based on outpatient settings in the USA and Canada, Sleath and colleagues (1999, 2000) investigated patient–physician communication about medication. Physicians and patients spent an average of 20% of each medical visit discussing medications. Almost half of the patients did not ask any medication questions at all, even though they were currently taking at least one medication. Starting a new medication doubled a patient's likelihood of question-asking (Sleath *et al.*, 1999). A fifth of patients expressed complaints about their medication and those who did so were twice as likely to express an adherence problem than patients who did not express a complaint (Sleath *et al.*, 2000).

Although it is likely that there will always be a proportion of patients who will prefer a more passive role in the consultation, and that these wishes must be respected, the option of involvement should be offered wherever practical (Coulter, 2002). There is evidence that older, less well-educated, those with more severe conditions and male patients may prefer a more paternalistic relationship with their doctor (Benbassat *et al.*, 1998). However, while many cancer patients may wish for the doctor to take a leading role, particularly in the earlier or acute stages of their illness, some cancer patients clearly prefer a greater level of involvement in treatment decision-making than they receive (Degner *et al.*, 1997). Equally, an older patient may not always want a paternalistic relationship. Kennelly and Bowling (2001) found that, amongst older patients with coronary heart disease, patients were frequently dissatisfied because of the lack of information about treatment options provided to them and the lack of opportunity to participate in decisions. These patients felt this implied a lack of respect for their views (Kennelly and Bowling, 2001). There is no accurate way, based on demographic factors alone, to predict which patients are more likely to prefer a paternalistic relationship. Patients' preferences may change over time, with the nature and severity of their condition and in the light of experience with effective patient participation (Coulter and Elwyn, 2002). Equally, evidence suggests that doctors are frequently unable to accurately 'guess' the level of information patients desire or their preference for role involvement (Strull *et al.*, 1984). The message seems quite clear. The only way to determine patients' preferences for information and their desired level of involvement in the consultation is to ask them.

Some researchers have analysed consultation transcripts in order to understand communication about medication in more detail. Smith-Dupre and Beck (1996) analysed the consultations of a single physician in which patient involvement was facilitated. The physician used self-disclosure as a way of downplaying perceived status differences and facilitating a cooperative approach. This enabled her patients to express their preferences about prescribed medication in the context of non-antagonistic consultations. In another study, Gwyn and Elwyn (1999) analysed a single consultation between the parents of a child with tonsillitis for whom antibiotics were not prescribed and a GP who regularly employed shared decision-making. In this consultation, the GP's efforts to reach a shared decision were thwarted by a combination of the embedded power imbalance and the conflict between the GP's and the parents' prescription preferences.

Few of the studies of communication about medicines have examined differences in patients' and doctors' perspectives, perhaps because this is rarely addressed in clinical practice. Pollock (2001), using a detailed case study, demonstrated how the lack of professional awareness of patients' ideas about illness and treatment can limit the capacity to provide effective healthcare. It can also reduce patients' ability to cope with their illness or to participate constructively in the management of disease.

What are the benefits of a concordant approach?

A fundamental question remains as to the impact of concordance on patient outcomes. To date, there has been little research exploring this issue specifically in relation to concordance. Reasons for this and a suggested strategy for future research are discussed in Chapter 7. A review by Lewin *et al.* (2002) examined the relationship between interventions for providers to promote a patient-centred approach and subsequent patient healthcare behaviours or health status. These reviewers defined patient-centred care as a philosophy of care that encourages shared control of the consultation, to include decisions about interventions or management, and a focus in the consultation on the patient as a whole person who has individual preferences situated within social contexts. These authors concluded that interventions to promote patient-centred care did improve the patient-centredness of the consultation process. Such consultation process indicators could include an increased display of empathic and facilitative responses, more psychosocial talk and a greater likelihood of the patient's concerns being addressed. Further, the reviewers found some evidence that these interventions improved patient satisfaction with care, although there was limited evidence that such interventions improved patient health status or healthcare behaviours such as adherence (Lewin *et al.*, 2002).

Stewart and colleagues (2000), in their review of the impact of patient-centred care on outcomes, concluded that patient-centred communication, as measured on their 'finding common ground' scale, was associated with better recovery from discomfort and concern, better emotional health and fewer diagnostic tests and referrals. There is some evidence to suggest that patients with chronic disease who are given more detailed information and who are 'coached' in a more participatory decision-making style will have better health outcomes, as measured by improved blood pressure or blood sugar control (Greenfield *et al.*, 1988; Kaplan *et al.*, 1989).

None the less, the true impact of concordance, particularly with regard to patient health outcomes, has yet to be fully elucidated. A recent systematic review of the literature relevant to concordance identified nine interventions involving two-way communications between health professionals and patients about medicines (Cox *et al.*, 2004). None of the interventions identified was based on the model of concordance and the fact that the interventions involved two-way communication does not necessarily mean that they used a concordant approach. However, many of the interventions did contain elements of concordance, such as encouraging patients to discuss their attitudes towards, and concerns about, medicines; addressing issues raised by patients; and working together with patients to develop a treatment regimen. The findings indicated that two-way communication between patients and professionals about medicine led to improved satisfaction with care, knowledge of their condition and treatment, adherence, and health outcomes and fewer medication-related problems.

Controversies, challenges and caveats

The sentence in the original definition of concordance, which stimulated the greatest debate and misinterpretation, is the last one:

> Although reciprocal, this is an alliance in which the most important determinations are agreed to be those that are made by the patient (Royal Pharmaceutical Society of Great Britain, 1997).

Although it refers to patient autonomy, it also reflects the pragmatic observation that consumers make their own decisions on a day-to-day basis about when, where and how to take their medicines. Unless the patient is closely supervised in hospital or undergoing directly observed treatment, healthcare practitioners cannot force people to take medicines against their will. They can deny access to medicines that patients want or that practitioners think unnecessary or harmful (for example, antibiotics). The point of concordance is to bring about awareness of any differences in patients' and practitioners' perspectives so that these can be discussed and negotiated. The outcome of a concordant consultation may be the agreement to differ.

In the recent discussion paper produced by the British Medical Association, one of the personal barriers to effective communication was described as doctors' lack of skill and understanding of the structures of conversational interaction (British Medical Association Board of Medical Education, 2003). This includes the use of clear and simple language, giving structured explanations and listening to patients' views. Doctors also describe a lack of some of the skills needed for the critical appraisal of information, to understand statistical information and in their ability to explain complex medical information to patients (Ford *et al.*, 2002). It would appear that providing healthcare professionals with the appropriate skills is essential to ensure the widespread implementation of concordance.

A number of criticisms have been made of the concept of concordance. Firstly, many practitioners fear that discussion of patients' views will lead to inordinately long consultations. However there is some evidence that discussion of patients' views does not necessarily lead to longer consultations (Belle Brown, 2003) and may in any case save time in the longer term through resolution of misunderstandings. Stewart and colleagues (1989) have suggested that physicians who are struggling with a patient-centred approach, but not fully utilising it, may need longer consultations but that this reduces as a physician masters the approach. In the Greenfield *et al.* study (1988), which linked greater patient participation in the consultation with improved health outcomes, although the total volume of talk in the intervention group was greater than that in the control group, there was no difference between them in terms of consultation length. Comparable results were reported by Marvel *et al.* (1999), who found that patients allowed to complete their statement of concerns used only 6 seconds more on average than those who were redirected before completion of concerns occurred. However, this American study had a mean consultation length of 15 minutes. Conversely, Howie *et al.* (1991) demonstrated an association between a positive response to the question 'Did the doctor give you a chance to say what was really on your mind?' and longer consultations. Time is a key issue and one which has been raised as a concern by healthcare professionals when discussing barriers to implementing shared decision-making (Elwyn *et al.*, 1999) and evidence-based patient choice (Ford *et al.*, 2002). It should be noted that time was a concern not only in relation to consultation length but also in the time needed to access information.

Some see concordance as a way of giving in to patients' inappropriate 'demands', or fear the medicolegal consequences of inappropriate prescribing. It is claimed by some that concordance shifts responsibility on to the patient or alternatively that it privileges patient autonomy. The model of concordance emphasises the importance of prescribers explaining their views as much as the converse, including the reasons why some prescriptions are seen as inappropriate by professionals. If some of the resistance to concordance is fuelled by reluctance to provide patients with sufficient information about their medicines, then this should be challenged. Medicolegal issues are likely to be particularly relevant in a small number of cases where patients refuse to take potentially life-saving medicines. In these cases, a concordant consultation would bring the patient's reluctance to the prescriber's attention. In a non-concordant consultation, the patient would leave without revealing his or her intentions not to take the medicine. Thus the point of concordance is not necessarily to change patients' behaviour, but to bring these differences into the open for discussion and negotiation. Medicolegally, all that has happened is that the prescriber is aware of something that he or she was previously unaware of. Such discussions should be recorded in patients' records to assist continuity of care and to document the advice given by the prescriber. Although prescribers may be concerned about the medicolegal repercussions of such an approach, evidence would suggest that good communication in the consultation is likely to lead to fewer malpractice claims. Levinson *et al.* (1997) classified physicians according to those who had no previous malpractice claims with those who had two or more claims and explored their communication behaviours. 'No-claims' physicians used more facilitative talk, such as soliciting patients' opinions and encouraging them to talk, than physicians with two or more malpractice claims. In an analysis of depositions in malpractice cases by Beckman *et al.* (1994), four types of communication problems were identified: deserting the patient, devaluing patients' views, delivering information poorly and failing to understand the patient's perspective. Concordance does not necessarily shift responsibility on to patients, as an exchange of views is relevant whoever takes the final responsibility for decision-making. Concordance brings greater transparency to this process and, if done well, is likely to lead to fewer medicolegal problems rather than more.

A final concern is that concordance could increase patient demand for more and more healthcare resources. While the evidence for this remains equivocal, there is some research to suggest that concordance could have the opposite effect. Decision aids are tools to facilitate patient involvement in decisions about their healthcare and can come in a number of different forms, frequently as an information booklet or video with worksheet. They can be seen as one way of operationalising the principles of shared decision-making and, potentially, concordance. A recent Cochrane review on decision aids (O'Connor *et al.*, 2002) suggests that people who are given a decision aid and involved in decision-making are more likely to go for more conservative options (e.g. watchful waiting) rather than surgery. In addition, this review revealed that decision aids increase knowledge, lower the uncertainty surrounding the decision-making process and allow more active patient participation in decision-making. The increasing use of technology and greater patient access to such information should facilitate the development of further decision aids covering a broad range of clinical conditions and, ideally, the process of greater patient involvement and concordance.

The way forward

The concept of concordance had its origins in a review of the problems associated with non-compliance, and for that reason is perhaps often confused with compliance. Unlike other models of the patient–professional relationship, it is focused on the processes involved in prescribing and taking medicines. The literature suggests that concordance is not being practised to any great extent, that a lack of concordance is associated with negative outcomes, and that two-way communication about medicines does lead to improved outcomes. Given the similarities between concordance and shared decision-making, the best way forward would seem to be greater collaboration between these two approaches so that the energies of practitioners, teachers and researchers in these two fields can be harnessed to best effect. While the writing of a prescription is still the most common outcome of many healthcare consultations, the focus on medicines is clearly a central issue for many patients and practitioners. However, communication about prescribing and medicines is part of a much wider context, with which those who are interested in concordance need to engage.

References

Beckman H B, Frankel R M (1984). The effect of physician behavior on the collection of data. *Ann Intern Med* 101: 692–696.

Beckman H B, Markakis K M, Suchman A L, Frankel R M (1994). The doctor–patient relationship and malpractice: lessons from plaintiff depositions. *Arch Intern Med* 154: 1365–1370.

Belle Brown J (2003). Time and the consultation. In: Jones R, Britten N, Culpepper L *et al.* (eds) *Oxford Textbook of Primary Medical Care*. Oxford: Oxford University Press, 190–193.

Benbassat J, Pilpel D, Tidhar M (1998). Patients' preferences for participation in clinical decision making: a review of published surveys. *Behav Med* 24: 81–88.

Braddock C L, Edwards K A, Hasenberg N M *et al.* (1999). Informed decision making in outpatient practice – time to get back to basics. *JAMA* 282: 2313–2320.

British Medical Association Board of Medical Education (2003). *Communication Skills Education for Doctors: A Discussion Paper*. London: BMA.

Britten N (2003). Clinicians' and patients' roles in patient involvement. *Qual Safe Health Care* 12: 87.

Britten N, Stevenson F A, Barry C A *et al.* (2000). Misunderstandings in prescribing decisions in general practice: qualitative study. *BMJ* 320: 484–488.

Campion P, Foulkes J, Neighbour R, Tate P (2002). Patient-centredness in the MRCGP video examination: analysis of large cohort. *BMJ* 325: 691–692.

Charles C, Gafni A, Whelan T (1997). Shared decision making in the medical encounter: what does it mean? (Or it takes at least two to tango.) *Soc Sci Med* 44: 681–692.

Charles C, Gafni A, Whelan T (1999). Decision making in the physician–patient encounter: revisiting the shared treatment decision-making model. *Soc Sci Med* 49: 651–661.

Coulter A (2002). *The Autonomous Patient – Ending Paternalism in Medical Care*. London: The John Fry Fellowship, The Nuffield Trust, The Stationery Office.

Coulter A, Elwyn G (2002). What do patients want from high-quality general practice and how do we involve them in improvement? *Br J Gen Pract* 52 (suppl): S22–S26.

Cox K, Stevenson F, Britten N, Dundar Y (2004). *A Systematic Review of Communication Between Patients and Health Care Professionals About Medicine-Taking and Prescribing*. London: Medicines Partnership.

Degner L F, Kristjanson L J, Bowman D *et al.* (1997). Information needs and decisional preferences in women with breast cancer. *JAMA* 277: 1485–1492.

Elwyn G, Charles C (2001). Shared decision making: the principles and the competences. In: Edwards A, Elwyn G (eds) *Evidence-Based Patient Choice: Inevitable or Impossible?* Oxford: Oxford University Press, 118–143.

Elwyn G, Edwards A, Gwyn R, Grol R (1999). Towards a feasible model for shared decision making: focus group study with general practice registrars. *BMJ* 319: 753–756.

Elwyn G, Edwards A, Kinnersley P, Grol R (2000). Shared decision making and the concept of equipoise: the competences of involving patients in healthcare choices. *Br J Gen Pract* 50: 892–897.

Fairclough N (1989). *Language and Power*. Harlow, Essex: Longman Group.

Ford S, Schofield T, Hope T (2002). Barriers to the evidence-based patient choice (EBPC) consultation. *Patient Educ Couns* 47: 179–185.

Greenfield S, Kaplan S H, Ware J E *et al.* (1988). Patients' participation in medical care: effect on blood sugar control and quality of life in diabetes. *J Gen Intern Med* 3: 448–457.

Gwyn R, Elwyn G (1999). When is a shared decision not (quite) a shared decision? Negotiating preferences in a general practice encounter. *Soc Sci Med* 49: 437–447.

Haynes R B, Montague P, Oliver T *et al.* (2001). *Interventions for Helping Patients to Follow Prescriptions for Medications* (Cochrane review). The Cochrane Library, issue 1. Oxford: Update Software.

Holmes-Rovner M, Llewellyn-Thomas H, Entwistle V *et al.* (2001). Patient choice modules for summaries of clinical effectiveness: a proposal. *BMJ* 322: 664–667.

Hope T (1996). *Evidence-Based Patient Choice*. London: King's Fund.

Howie J G R, Porter A M D, Heaney D J, Hopton J L (1991). Long to short consultation ratio: a proxy measure of quality of care for general practice. *Br J Gen Pract* 41: 48–54.

Kaplan S H, Greenfield S, Ware J E (1989). Assessing the effects of physician–patient interactions on the outcomes of chronic disease. *Med Care* 27 (suppl.): S110–S127.

Katon W, Kleinman A (1981). Doctor–patient negotiation and other social science strategies in patient care. In: Eisenberg L, Kleinman A (ed) *The Relevance of Social Science for Medicine*, pp. 253–279. Dordrecht, Netherlands: D. Reidel.

Kennelly C, Bowling A (2001). Suffering in deference: a focus group study of older cardiac patients' preferences for treatment and perceptions of risk. *Qual Health Care* 10 (suppl. 1): i23–i28.

Kjellgren K I, Svensson S, Ahlner J, Saljo R (1998). Antihypertensive medication in clinical encounters. *Int J Cardiol* 64: 161–169.

Kjellgren K I, Svensson S, Ahlner J, Saljo R (2000). Antihypertensive treatment and patient autonomy – the follow-up appointment as a resource for care. *Patient Educ Couns* 40: 39–49.

Levinson W, Roter D L, Mullooly J P *et al.* (1997). Physician–patient communication – the relationship with malpractice claims among primary care physicians and surgeons. *JAMA* 277: 553–559.

Lewin S A, Skea Z C, Entwistle V *et al.* (2002). *Interventions for Providers to Promote a Patient-Centred Approach in Clinical Consultations* (Cochrane review). The Cochrane Library, issue 4. Oxford: Update Software.

Makoul G, Arntson P, Schofield T (1995). Health promotion in primary care: physician–patient communication and decision making about prescription medications. *Soc Sci Med* 41: 1241–1254.

Marvel H K, Epstein R M, Flowers K, Beckman H B (1999). Soliciting the patient's agenda – have we improved? *JAMA* 281: 283–287.

Mead N, Bower P (2000). Patient-centredness: a conceptual framework and review of the empirical literature. *Soc Sci Med* 51: 1087–1110.

O'Connor A M, Stacey D, Rovner D *et al.* (2002). *Decision Aids for People Facing Health Treatment or Screening Decisions* (Cochrane review). The Cochrane Library, issue 2. Oxford: Update Software.

Pollock K (2001). 'I've not asked him, you see, and he's not said': understanding lay explanatory models of illness is a prerequisite for concordant consultations. *Int J Pharm Pract* 9: 105–117.

Roter D L, Hall J A (1992). *Doctors Talking to Patients, Patients Talking to Doctors: Improving Communication in Medical Visits.* Westport, CT: Auburn House.

Royal Pharmaceutical Society of Great Britain (1997). *From Compliance to Concordance: Achieving Shared Goals in Medicine Taking.* London: RPSGB.

Silverman J D, Kurtz S M, Draper J (1998). *Skills for Communicating with Patients.* Oxford: Radcliffe Medical Press.

Sleath B, Roter D, Chewning B, Svarstad B (1999). Asking questions about medication: analysis of physician–patient interactions and physician perceptions. *Med Care* 37: 1169–1173.

Sleath B, Chewning B, Svarstad B, Roter D (2000). Patient expression of complaints and adherence problems with medications during chronic disease medical visits. *J Soc Admin Pharm* 17: 71–80.

Smith-Dupre A A, Beck C S (1996). Enabling patients and physicians to pursue multiple goals in health care encounters: a case study. *Health Commun* 8: 73–90.

Stevenson F A, Barry C A, Britten N *et al.* (2000). Doctor–patient communication about drugs: the evidence for shared decision making. *Soc Sci Med* 50: 829–840.

Stewart M (2001). Towards a global definition of patient-centred care. *BMJ* 322: 444–445.

Stewart M, Belle Brown J, Weston W W (1989). Patient-centred interviewing part III: five provocative questions. *Can Fam Phys* 35: 159–161.

Stewart M, Belle Brown J, Donner A *et al.* (2000). The impact of patient-centered care on outcomes. *J Fam Pract* 49: 796–804.

Stewart M, Belle Brown J, Wayne Weston W *et al.* (2003). *Patient-Centred Medicine: Transforming the Clinical Method*, 2nd edn. Abingdon: Radcliffe Medical Press.

Stimson G V (1974). Obeying doctor's orders: a view from the other side. *Soc Sci Med* 8: 97–104.

Strull W M, Lo B, Charles G (1984). Do patients want to participate in medical decision making? *JAMA* 252: 2990–2994.

Towle A, Godolphin W (1999). Framework for teaching and learning informed shared decision making. *BMJ* 319: 766–771.

Tuckett D, Boulton M, Olson C, Williams A (1985). *Meetings Between Experts: An Approach to Sharing Ideas in Medical Consultations.* London: Tavistock Publications.

Vernon G (2003). Immunisation policy: from compliance to concordance? *Br J Gen Pract* 53: 399–404.

3

The patient's perspective

Fiona Stevenson

Introduction

This chapter examines the basis for concordance and the evidence that supports it, focusing on the patient's perspective. Initially some key aspects of concordance, which are of particular relevance to the patient's perspective, are outlined. This is followed by an examination of the literature in five areas:

1. patients' beliefs about illness and medicines
2. the extent to which patients play an active role outside the consultation with particular reference to medicine-taking behaviour
3. communication between healthcare practitioners and patients in the consultation
4. the wider context within which prescribing and medicine-taking occur
5. the potential barriers to the implementation of concordance.

The chapter concludes by raising a number of issues that may require resolution in the future.

Key aspects of concordance

Concordance is based on the idea that healthcare practitioners and patients should work towards a mutual understanding in relation to medicine-taking and the development of a therapeutic alliance. Fundamental to the concept of concordance is that there is an open exchange of beliefs about medicines upon which both prescribing and medicine-taking decisions may then be based. Thus concordance seeks to make patient participation explicit.

The exchange of beliefs and views by both healthcare professionals and patients may result in an agreement to differ over treatment choices but the key issue is that all the participants in the consultation are aware of differences where they exist. This awareness may then be used as the basis for joint negotiation or compromise as to the final outcome. Thus concordance seeks to make apparent potential areas of disagreement and conflict. Indeed, Britten (2001) argued that the significance of the concept of concordance is that it acknowledges patients' autonomy and the potential conflict between patient and doctor.

The ideas which form the basis of the concordance model are not new; similar ideas can be found in literature published in the 1980s (e.g. Katon and Kleinman, 1981; Tuckett *et al.*, 1985). There are however two key ideas in relation to concordance from the patient's perspectives. Firstly, patients have specific beliefs about both their illness and their medicines which are central to their decision-making about medicine-taking, and secondly, the extent to which patients are prepared to take an active role in relation to their healthcare. These ideas are now explored in more detail.

Patients' beliefs about illness and medicine

Williams and Wood (1986) argued that it is necessary to recognise the place that lay beliefs occupy in a patient's life and thoughts. Lay explanations of illness affect illness appraisal, self-treatment, decisions to seek care and changes in daily regimens (Mechanic, 1992). Patients have complex sets of beliefs, drawn from their own and their families' experiences, and any advice that they are given has to pass through a filter of these beliefs. These beliefs may be internally consistent but often contradict biomedical theories (Donovan *et al.*, 1989). Pollock (2001) argued that an understanding of lay explanatory models of illness, as well as patients' views of medicine, is necessary for a concordant consultation. Moreover, a lack of professional awareness and understanding of patients' models of illness limits the capacity to provide effective healthcare and reduces patients' ability to cope with the experience of illness or to participate actively in the management of their disease (Pollock, 2001).

Britten (1996) pointed out that, compared with the extensive literature on lay beliefs about illness, the literature on lay views of drugs and medicines is sparse and is chiefly concerned with adherence to prescribed medicines. Drawing on a dataset of interviews with 30 adults, Britten distinguished between what she termed 'orthodox' and 'unorthodox' accounts of medicines. 'Orthodox' accounts were those in which patients gave a largely taken-for-granted, unquestioning account of their medicines, while 'unorthodox' accounts, which outnumbered the 'orthodox' accounts, contained within them descriptions of 'aversion' to medicines. Medicines were presented as 'unnatural' and 'damaging', and doctors were frequently criticised for overprescribing.

The people who held these views were not concerned about medical legitimisation of their views and therefore these accounts were not reported to be shared in the consultation. It will be difficult to achieve a concordant consultation with patients who hold such views if they do not perceive a need to share with medical practitioners.

The active role of patients outside the consultation

Concordance requires patients to take an active role in their medical care. The literature makes clear the ways in which patients play an active decision-making role both before and after consultations.

Before patients receive any medical care they actively have to make the decision to seek care based on a judgement that their symptoms require medical advice. As long ago as 1975, Bloor and Horobin discussed the phenomenon of the double bind, in which they explored the idea that doctors, especially GPs, operate with a contradictory view of patient behaviour. On the one hand the patient is supposed to be the well-informed citizen who knows when it is appropriate to consult the doctor. On the other hand, the same patient should 'defer to the opinion of the doctor' once in the consultation room (Bloor and Horobin, 1975). Concordance seeks to resolve this by making the patients' views about why they consulted relevant to the actual consultation, and incorporating patients' views into decisions about treatment.

Other research has demonstrated that patients make judgements about the result of a consultation some time after its completion, sometimes by recounting 'atrocity stories' (Stimson and Webb, 1975). Patients' active roles after the consultation are illustrated by the finding that up to 50% of people on medication for chronic diseases do not take their medicine in fully therapeutic doses (Sackett and Snow, 1979).

It is known that patients' beliefs about medicine affect their medicine-taking behaviour. Donovan and Blake's (1992) study of patients' reactions to advice about medications prescribed by doctors in rheumatology clinics showed that patients are not on the whole passive or powerless. Rather they are capable of making choices about treatments and lifestyles rationally within the context of their beliefs, responsibilities and preferences. Patients have many beliefs and theories that suggest courses of action; these are moderated by information from others, particularly family members, medical staff and the media (Stevenson et al., 1999). Pollock (2001) argued that professional judgement may be viewed merely as one among several different options for consideration by patients when considering medical advice and pre-scriptions.

Conrad (1985), based on research with people prescribed medica-tion for epilepsy, presented the idea that people may alter their medica-tion regimen in an attempt to assert some degree of control over their condition. This fits with the conclusion drawn by Donovan and Blake (1992), and Morgan (1996), that although non-compliance may be per-ceived as deviance from the perspective of the healthcare professional, when examined from the perspective of the patient it appears more as reasoned decision-making.

Donovan and Blake (1992) concluded that there should be a move away from the notion of compliance towards the incorporation of the patient's perspective:

> Perhaps the issue now should not be compliance, but how medical staff can understand and participate in the decisions that patients already take about their medications! (Donovan and Blake, 1992: 512)

This suggests a reverse in the balance of power between patients and medical practitioners to a position in which healthcare professionals contribute to patients' decisions. Arguably this statement goes further towards shifting the balance of power towards patients than the con-cordance model, which argues for patients and practitioners to parti-cipate as equal partners to reach an agreement on treatment.

Having discussed the active role of patients outside the consulta-tion, the role of patients inside the consultation is now discussed.

Communication between healthcare practitioners and patients in the consultation

Concordance requires both patients and healthcare professionals to be active in the consultation. A review of the literature by Stewart (1995) concluded that four key dimensions of communication were related to positive outcomes:

1. the provision of clear information
2. questions from the patient
3. willingness to share and discuss decisions
4. agreement between patients and doctors about both the problem and the plan

The case for incorporating patients' beliefs into clinical decision-making rests on claims that this will lead to improved satisfaction with the process of care and better health outcomes. Although much of the evidence for this comes from North America (Coulter, 1997), work in the UK has provided some support for these findings. For example, Barry and colleagues (2001) illustrated that increased attention to patients' contextually grounded experiences of events and problems in their life makes for better outcomes and more 'humane' care.

However, in many consultations there is little meaningful dialogue between GPs and patients about the nature of the problem and possible therapeutic actions (Tuckett *et al.*, 1985). Elwyn and colleagues (1999a), in their discussion of shared decision-making, suggested that communication skills development has focused on uncovering and matching agendas, with the effect that the 'second half' of the consultation, where decisions are made and future management agreed, has been neglected. They concluded that it is necessary to place more emphasis on the second part of the consultation. Yet arguably if agendas and information are not successfully shared in the first part of the consultation, then it will not be possible to achieve a shared decision about treatment.

The link between patient preferences for participation and actual participation is not very strong (Charles *et al.*, 1997), with consultations mainly being characterised by patient passivity and non-participation (Elwyn *et al.*, 1999a, 1999b). However, this does not mean that patients are totally passive in the consultation.

Although there is an increasing focus on the issue of patient participation, the classic text by Stimson and Webb (1975), published nearly 30 years ago, presented the argument that both doctors and patients employ strategies and negotiation tactics. Patients, for example, rehearse what they will say, partially present symptoms, exclude information and ignore the doctor's advice. In this sense patients are not merely passive partners in the process. Helman (1978) further extended the work of Stimson and Webb with his argument that any negotiation is further complicated by the fact that it is not just between two or more individuals but also between two systems of thought representing the professional and the patient perspective. Concordance seeks to bring together these two perspectives.

Work by Tuckett and colleagues (1985), published a decade after the work of Stimson and Webb (1975), reported that in at least half of the consultations they studied there was clear evidence of attempts by patients to influence the sharing of information. There is also a range of literature to suggest that, although professional–patient relationships are inherently unequal, both participants are able to influence the outcomes of consultations (Nettleton, 1995). Nettleton argued that the relationship between professionals and patients is likely to be enhanced if practitioners are able both to recognise and encourage the involvement of patients, while the importance of patients' assessments of consultations was highlighted by the work of Howie *et al.* (1998) on enablement. The evidence from all these studies supports the ideas that form the basis of the concordance initiative.

The wider context within which prescribing and medicine-taking occur

Having considered concordance at the level of individual interactions between patients and healthcare professionals, the chapter now moves on to consider the wider context within which these individual interactions take place.

The traditional model of medical decision-making in which doctors use their knowledge, skills and judgement to make decisions on behalf of their patients has come under increasing pressure in recent years (Coulter, 1997) with support for models such as patient-centred medicine (Stewart *et al.*, 1995) and shared decision-making (Charles *et al.*, 1997). These models have already been explored in detail in Chapter 2, but are included here as a link to the patient's agenda. Thus doctors can no longer rely on a paternalistic model of medical practice in which the patient will act as requested because of the position of authority of the doctor, but rather a persuasive model of the relationship is increasingly perceived to be more appropriate (Scambler and Britten, 2001).

Another driver for change has been the widespread media coverage of recent cases such as the Bristol Royal Infirmary and Alder Hey hospital organs retention scandal (BBC News Online 29/01/01), the inquiry into the treatment and care of babies undergoing complex heart surgery at the Bristol Royal Infirmary between 1983 and 1995 (Bristol Royal Infirmary Inquiry, 2001), as well as the case of Harold Shipman (Smith, 2001). These have raised awareness of the need for accountability and assurance of probity in the delivery of medical services rather than an assumed professional beneficence. Thus the position of trust of doctors in society may be seen as being challenged, and the rights of patients to have their views taken into account has become recognised.

Moreover, the growth of, and increasing ease of access to, medical information, together with the media interest in medical issues, the increasing use of alternative medicines and the growth of self-help groups all give credence to the idea that the position of the doctor as a central source of information and authority concerning illness and its treatment has shifted (Bury, 1997).

Thus, it has been suggested that:

> The doctor–patient relationship is changing rapidly towards a more active partnership, fostered by the increasing access to information about treatments and the consumerist trends in modern society (Elwyn *et al.*, 1999a).

All these changes indicate that, in situations where there are several treatment options with different possible outcomes, the case for incorporating patients' preferences into the decision-making process is strong.

Much of the discussion in this area focuses on the role of doctors; however, such changes also affect relationships with other healthcare professionals such as pharmacists and nurses. Although they are not generally involved in the actual act of prescribing, they have a key role in discussing medicine and issues concerning the use of medicines, particularly in relation to chronic illness. In addition the plans to widen the authority to prescribe (Department of Health, 2000) will make their professional role of increasing relevance in relation to concordance.

In addition to changes affecting the role of professionals, the nature of 'patienthood' has altered significantly in recent years. Not only has the population aged but also the increasing prevalence of chronic illness has been accompanied by a tendency for patients to be more knowledgeable about their condition. Thus, in the context of general practice, the patient may now become an 'expert' in situations in which the doctor may have only a general understanding of the disorder. The possibilities and constraints of a more 'shared' approach to care in such situations needs to be considered (Bury, 1997).

Patients are encouraged to take responsibility for their own health, to exercise choice and to act as discriminating 'consumers' (Nettleton, 1995). Giddens (1991) provided some useful insights into the changing nature of expertise. He argued that expanding expertise may lead both to the 'de-skilling' of lay people and the 'sequestration' of experience from everyday life, and also to a 'reskilling' in which people become active and 'empowered' (Giddens, 1991: 138). So while medical expertise may reduce patients' confidence in the face of illness, new forms of information and action (e.g. the internet or participating in self-help groups) may help them to restore a sense of control. Hardey's research, which examined the potential of the internet to change doctor–patient communication about treatment, provides an illustration of how technology may give patients control over their healthcare. In particular he discussed not only the availability of information, but also that patients were 'empowered' by the fact that they control what and how much information they collect (Hardey, 1999).

Following on from the evidence-based healthcare movement, the notion of evidence-based patient choice has been developed. Entwistle and O'Donnell (2001) argued that the potential of evidence-based approaches to improve the quality of healthcare decisions will be enhanced if patients are appropriately involved in identifying the questions that need to be asked and in considering the implications of the available research evidence for their own healthcare choices. Thus once again the active involvement of patients in their own healthcare is advocated.

This shift in emphasis away from paternalism is also apparent in health policy. The policy of involving patients in their healthcare decisions has been evident in the form of *The Patients' Charter* since 1991 (Department of Health, 1991) and continued with *Patient Partnership: Building a Collaborative Strategy* in 1996, which emphasised the intention to 'promote user involvement in their own care, as active partners with professionals' (NHS Executive, 1996). A similar focus is also present in *The NHS Plan* (Department of Health, 2000) which outlined plans to make the health service more patient-centred, while the report outlining the Expert Patient initiative suggested that there is a new emphasis on the relationship between the NHS and the people it serves – one in which health professionals and patients are genuine partners seeking together the best solutions to each patient's problem, and that patients should be empowered with information and contribute ideas to help in their treatment and care without fear of intimidation or ridicule (Department of Health, 2001).

In addition to the publication of policy documents, the promotion of programmes such as the Medicines Partnership (www.medicines-partnership.org) and the Expert Patient (Department of Health, 2001) programmes provide just two examples of the ways in which the role of the patient is being presented by the government as central to any treatment. Both suggest that the knowledge and experience held by the patient has for too long been an untapped resource.

The Medicines Partnership programme seeks to examine the possibilities for the implementation of ongoing research findings on concordance through the Task Force on Medicines Partnership. It has two overall aims: to achieve greater health benefit for patients and to improve patient satisfaction with the delivery of healthcare. The work is based on three core principles:

1. The patient should be seen as a partner and actively participate in treatment.
2. When drug treatment is being prescribed or monitored, patients are asked about their experience of and attitude to the disease and its treatment, and that the prescriber ascertains that the patient knows how and why prescribed medicines should be used.
3. Professionals work as partners to improve the patients' active participation in the treatment.

In summary, the views and experiences of patients are presented as central to their treatment.

The Expert Patient programme is based on the idea that people with chronic conditions are often in the best position to know what they need in terms of managing their own condition, yet recognises that the process may be impeded by professional attitudes, skills and time and by patients' attitudes and skills. The solution is presented as the development of user-led self-management programmes. It is argued that today's patients with chronic diseases need not be mere recipients of care: they can become key decision-makers in the treatment process (Department of Health, 2001). The report continues:

> By ensuring that knowledge of their condition is developed to a point where they are empowered to take some responsibility for its management and work in partnership with their health and social care providers, patients can be given greater control over their lives (Department of Health, 2001).

Yet, much as this document provides support for the role of active patients, the role of the active patient appears to be sanctioned only so long as it fits with the views of health and social care providers. Thus, despite the concept of the Expert Patient being based on the idea that patients are already knowledgeable, the report suggests that this knowledge should be developed to a level whereby self-management, within the bounds of a medical regimen, becomes a real option. What is unclear is the status of patients' own knowledge, which may contradict the biomedical knowledge held by healthcare professionals. There is no discussion of patients' experiential knowledge being directly shared; rather, patients' knowledge is incorporated into a structured programme. This is one of the key differences between the Expert Patient programme and concordance as advocated by Medicines Partnership. The Expert Patient initiative is based on the creation of a cadre of expert patients – people who have the confidence, skills, information and knowledge to play a central role in the management of life with chronic diseases in order to minimise the impact of disease on their lives. Concordance, in contrast, rather than focusing on creating an 'expert' patient, is based on the assumption that patients already possess expertise which should be directly shared with healthcare professionals so that they can work together towards a partnership. Thus, although the Expert Patient initiative presents a promise of sharing of professional power, professional and patient expertise do not appear to be seen as different but equal in the same way as they are in the concordance model. A final, and key, difference between concordance and the Expert Patient initiative is that the latter is only concerned with chronic illness and makes no reference to patient expertise around acute illness.

Potential barriers to concordance

Despite all the evidence to suggest that patients may be in a position to embrace concordance, or at least elements of it, the literature, in particular that concerned with communication between doctors and patients, indicates that there are currently a number of potential barriers to the implementation of concordance.

Discussions during consultations of patients' opinions about medicines are vital for understanding non-adherence (Donovan and Blake, 1992; Britten, 1994) and a necessary component of concordance, yet are rare (Makoul et al., 1995). In a study involving 20 doctors and 62 patients, none of the doctors appeared to have a clear idea of any of the patients' views about medicine (Stevenson et al., 2000). Moreover, Tuckett et al. (1985) reported that doctors' behaviour in the consultation did not appear to involve active negotiation with patients, and doctors rarely asked about or responded to patients' ideas. The same authors also suggested that patients do not share their ideas in the consultation for fear of making it uncomfortable and tense (Tuckett et al., 1985).

If patients are to be able to take part in concordant consultations then they need to feel comfortable about sharing their agendas with the doctor, yet research suggests that this is not the case and people rarely express all their agenda items. In particular, agenda items relating to theories or worries about diagnosis and not wanting a prescription are not always raised (Barry et al., 2000). Failure to share agendas may not only cause problems in terms of achieving concordance but has been shown to have an actual, or potential, effect on medicines-taking behaviour (Britten et al., 2000).

Although sharing of information is necessary as a basis for sharing decisions, sharing information and sharing decisions are not synonymous (Ong *et al.*, 1995). An analysis of 62 consultations with GPs who were interested in communication in the consultation concluded that not only could the decisions made in those consultations not be termed shared decision-making, but also that sharing of information at even a basic level was not happening (Stevenson *et al.*, 2000). In addition, what appeared on the surface to be a consultation that gave precedence to the patient's opinions of management, on closer examination appeared rather closer to an abdication of responsibility on the part of the GP, leaving the patient unsure about the final decision. This demonstrates the necessity of examining consultation behaviour in detail before making any judgements about what is happening in the consultation.

Research has mainly focused on the role of healthcare professionals and how they need to change their practice to be more 'patient-centred'. Stewart and Brown (2001) argued that patient-centred medicine requires a shift in the mindset of the clinician away from the historical hierarchical notion of a professional in charge with a passive patient, to a situation in which power is shared. The adoption of a model such as concordance is reliant on the cooperation of healthcare professionals, as even if patients wish to be involved in a discussion of their symptoms and treatment, this can be blocked by the doctor. This was demonstrated by Barry and colleagues (2001), who provided examples of instances in which patients' attempts to discuss their concerns or medical problems in relation to their everyday lives were either 'blocked' by doctors or ignored.

Pollock (2001) argued, based on her extended analysis of a single case, that even if the GP in her analysis had been aware that his patient harboured such a complex explanatory model of her illness, and of her associated anxiety, it is unlikely that any attempt on his part to uncover and discuss these anxieties would have met with much success. Pollock (2001) pointed out that the patient felt too inhibited, shamefaced and time-pressured in the consulting room to be comfortable about disclosing her thoughts and feelings, although outside the surgery she applied a well-developed capacity for theorising and critical reflection. This suggests that, although researchers have documented patients' knowledge, beliefs and opinions about their medical problems and their medicines, these may not be available to the doctor in the consultation if the patient does not judge this to be appropriate. Thus we have to remain aware of both the explicit and implicit structural constraints of the healthcare system.

Pollock (2001) draws on the work of Strong (1979) and his notion of the 'bureaucratic format' to note that consultations are disciplined and constrained against the exchange of information necessary for concordance. She discussed the role of doctors' training and the emphasis on disease (organic pathology) as opposed to illness (the patient's subjective experience of symptoms). She stated:

> Where both doctors and patients remain constrained by the etiquette of the bureaucratic format to take what is said merely at face value, it is less likely that patient understanding and concerns will be aired, explored or shared in the course of achieving a genuinely negotiated outcome (Pollock, 2001).

The challenges for moving forward

The challenges for the future of concordance from the patient's perspective may be seen to fall into three main areas:

1. the acceptability and feasibility of concordance from the patient's perspective
2. the rights and responsibilities of both patients and practitioners in relation to concordance
3. practical issues in relation to the implementation and assessment of whether or not concordance is being achieved

These are each discussed in more detail below.

The acceptability and feasibility of concordance

Research is needed on both the acceptability and feasibility of concordance from the perspective of all the stakeholders: patients, healthcare professionals and policy-makers. Even if concordance is judged to be both acceptable and feasible, there are still questions, such as, can people 'opt out' of concordance, and if so, to what extent? Moreover, given that preferences for participation are likely to vary according to the presenting problem, are patients prepared to renegotiate their role in each consultation?

A prescription is a visible token of the social relationship between patients and practitioners (Hall, 1980) and therefore discussions that may result in the rejection of a prescription, which is a possible outcome of a concordant consultation, may be particularly difficult for patients for fear this may be perceived as a rejection of the doctor.

Concordance, in part, draws on a model of an informed patient. However, although there has been an increase in the availability of information, it is not necessarily equally available, as access to books and resources such as the internet is not equally distributed. There may also be an issue of literacy and language, particularly for people from minority ethnic groups. It may be that the well informed are becoming better informed while the less well informed remain in this state.

Concordance relies on the participation of both healthcare professionals and patients, therefore a lack of commitment on the part of either party will make a concordant consultation impossible. This should not be taken to imply that patients have to participate in medical decision-making for concordance to be achieved, but rather patients have to have had the opportunity to be involved even if they wish decisions to be taken on their behalf. Conversely, one of the concerns expressed by healthcare professionals in relation to concordance is that patients may 'demand' a particular treatment which is not indicated on grounds of either or both clinical- or cost-effectiveness. Instead, the notion of concordance stresses the need for sharing of knowledge and expertise on the part of both patients and professionals and therefore prescribing a treatment which is not indicated would not be judged to form part of a concordant consultation as this would suggest that professional expertise had not been taken account of in the decision-making process.

It is important to consider whether patients' perceptions of the possibility of achieving concordance varies according to the healthcare professional involved. For example, is it perceived by patients to be more feasible with some professionals than others? Does it depend on personalities? As a postscript to her chapter on narrative and patient choice, Greenhalgh (2001) reflects on the effect of the relationship with the patient, suggesting that the ease with which shared decisions may be accomplished is likely to vary according to the interpersonal dynamics between the patient and the professional. At the extreme, it is difficult for people to seek a greater involvement if they do not perceive this to be a possibility or an option.

Shared decision-making is not the same as concordance; however, it shares similar principles. Coulter (1997) pointed out that concerns about shared decision-making come from a number of quarters: from clinicians anxious about losing their autonomy, from patients' advocates worried about the adverse effects of information and from policy-makers worried about the impact on costs and equity. This general resistance to shared decision-making indicates that practitioners, patients and policy-makers may all need to be persuaded of the advantages of concordance and have any concerns allayed before it will be possible to implement it in practice.

Finally, it is important to consider whose agenda concordance represents. The concept originated from a working party of academics and clinicians with a focus on a 'medical' problem: 'Why don't people take their medicine as directed?' The issue from the patient's point of view, following Donovan (1995), is that patients do not necessarily see their behaviour as a problem, but rather as reasoned decision-making. This potential mismatch between patients and practitioners needs to be addressed if concordance is to be achieved in practice.

The rights and responsibilities of patients and practitioners

The effects for patients of concordant consultations in terms of increased rights and responsibilities for their treatment cannot be ignored. In return for an increased voice in consultations they need to be prepared to accept increased responsibility for the decisions made. This once again raises the issue of the acceptability of concordance to patients. Both Elwyn *et al.* (1999a) and Donovan and Blake (1992) provide useful summaries of the rights and responsibilities of professionals and patients with regard to sharing decisions in the consultation.

Elwyn *et al.* (1999a) argued that the clinician should be prepared to adapt to the patient's preferred role, and therefore to hand over, share or take overall responsibility for decision-making. In relation to the patient, they argued that involvement would bring new responsibilities, in particular a requirement to evaluate risks and benefits. Following their consideration of people's medicine-taking behaviour, Donovan and Blake (1992) argued that the development of active, cooperative relationships between patients and doctors requires recognition on the part of doctors of patients' decision-making abilities, development of an understanding of patients' needs and constraints and a commitment to work with patients in the development of treatment regimens. For their part patients will need to be more explicit about their needs and expectations, particularly how they reach their decisions about treatments.

Practical issues in relation to implementation and assessment

In terms of the implementation of concordance, it is worth reflecting on the lessons that can be drawn from the Expert Patient programme. The

Expert Patient programme makes a distinction between sufferers of acute and chronic conditions. Should this distinction also be made in relation to concordance? Holman and Lorig (2000) suggested that, when acute illnesses were the primary cause of ill health, patients were inexperienced and passive. Now that chronic illnesses are more prevalent they suggest that patients must become partners in treatment and that this should have benefits not just for the patient but also in terms of the wider goals of efficiency and efficacy. Should this be taken further to suggest that concordance is better-suited to chronic problems, as opposed to acute illnesses? It is possible that concordance fits better with chronic illness for both the patient and the doctor. Thus patients have time to consider their symptoms and possible treatments, while for the doctors chronic illnesses may give them the opportunity to develop an understanding of the patient's perspective over a number of consultations. Perhaps chronic problems should be seen as the starting point for the development of means by which concordance can be implemented in practice?

The practical issue of how concordance can be measured produces similar issues to the arguments raised in relation to the measurement of shared decision-making (Stevenson *et al.*, 2000). This is covered in more detail in Chapter 7. Stevenson *et al.* (2000) argued, in relation to the measurement of shared decision-making, that further consideration is required to determine what is meant by agreement and consensus, and how valid assessment and measurement of these may be achieved. It is also necessary to recognise the differential knowledge and resources that doctors and patients bring to consultations, and the notion that doctors may 'frame' any information provided to favour certain options.

The issue of framing was clearly illustrated by Silverman (1987). Using data drawn from audio recordings of a paediatric cardiology clinic, he argued that the consultation normally involves attempts by physicians to supplant parents' social discourse by a clinical discourse. In contrast, in clinics attended by parents of children with Down's syndrome, the doctors conspired with parents to supplant a clinical language by a social discourse that depicted the child's present enjoyment of life within an idealised family setting. This allowed the doctor to argue effectively against medical interventions. Conversely, references to the medical world were used to encourage parents with children with similar heart problems but without Down's syndrome to agree to a surgical intervention. Thus Silverman notes the power of the 'framing' of information and the potentially coercive nature of the way in which information is provided. In terms of concordance there is also another message. Reference to the social world, or to what Mishler (1984) refers to as the 'lifeworld', may be coercive and oppressive. It is therefore necessary to consider the extent to which it is possible to enter the patient's world without it being perceived as an extension of medical power. There is a balance to achieve, such that the inclusion of patients' views and opinions in a consultation are perceived as part of a move towards partnership and not as a means of coercion. This of course has implications in terms of measuring the existence or otherwise of concordance in consultations.

Conclusion

This chapter has outlined the evidence relating to the model of concordance in terms of the suggestion that patients are in a position to embrace concordance, or at least elements of it, and the potential barriers to, and likely challenges in working towards, implementation. It has also highlighted the need for research to assess the acceptability of concordance from the perspective of all the stakeholders, including patients.

The changes in the wider social and political climate and within health service organisation that are outlined in this chapter have not yet been reflected in medical consultations, which largely consist of patient passivity and non-participation (Elwyn et al., 1999a, 1999b). If concordance is to succeed it requires the commitment of both patients and healthcare professionals. However, given the continuing imbalance of power relations in consultations, it is arguably the responsibility of the healthcare professional to take the initiative in this.

References

Barry C A, Bradley C P, Britten N et al. (2000). Patients' unvoiced agendas in general practice consultations: qualitative study. *BMJ* 320: 1246–1250.

Barry C A, Stevenson F, Britten N et al. (2001). Giving voice to the lifeworld. More humane, more effective medical care? *Soc Sci Med* 53: 487–505.

Bloor M, Horobin G (1975). Conflict and conflict resolution in doctor/patient interactions. In: Cox C, Mead A (eds) *A Sociology of Medical Practice*. London: Collier-Macmillan, 271–284.

Bristol Royal Infirmary Inquiry (2001). Learning from Bristol: The Report of the Public Inquiry into Children's Heart Surgery at the Bristol Royal Infirmary 1984–1995. London: Stationery Office. Available online at: www.bristol-inquiry.org.uk (accessed 5 April 2004).

Britten N (1994). Patients' ideas about medicines: a qualitative study in a general practice population. *Br J Gen Pract* 44: 465–468.

Britten N (1996). Lay views of drugs and medicines: orthodox and unorthodox accounts. In: Williams S J, Calnan M (eds) *Modern Medicines: Lay Perspectives and Experiences*. London: UCL Press, 48–73.

Britten N (2001). Prescribing and the defense of clinical autonomy. *Sociol Health Illness* 23: 478–496.

Britten N, Stevenson F A, Barry C A *et al.* (2000). Misunderstandings in prescribing decisions in general practice: qualitative study. *BMJ* 320: 484–488.

Bury M (1997). *Health and Illness in a Changing Society*. London: Routledge.

Charles C, Gafni A, Whelan T (1997). Shared decision-making in the medical encounter: what does it mean? (Or it takes at least two to tango.) *Soc Sci Med* 44: 681–692.

Conrad P (1985). The meaning of medications: another look at compliance. *Soc Sci Med* 20: 29–37.

Coulter A (1997). Partnership with patients: the pros and cons of shared clinical decision-making. *J Health Serv Res Policy* 2: 112–121.

Department of Health (1991). *The Patients' Charter*. London: HMSO.

Department of Health (2000). *The NHS Plan. A Plan for Investment. A Plan for Reform*. London: HMSO.

Department of Health (2001). *The Expert Patient: A New Approach to Chronic Disease Management for the 21st Century*. London: Department of Health.

Donovan J L (1995). Patient decision making. The missing ingredient in compliance research. *Int J Technol Assess Health Care* 11: 443–455.

Donovan J L, Blake D R (1992). Patient non-compliance: deviance or reasoned decision making? *Soc Sci Med* 34: 507–513.

Donovan J L, Blake D R, Fleming W G (1989). The patient is not a blank sheet: lay beliefs and their relevance to patient education. *Br J Rheumatol* 28: 58–61.

Elwyn G, Edwards A, Kinnersley P (1999a). Shared decision-making in primary care: the neglected second half of the consultation. *Br J Gen Pract* 49: 477–482.

Elwyn G, Edwards A, Gwyn R, Grol R (1999b). Towards a feasible model for shared decision making: focus group study with general practice registrars. *BMJ* 319: 753–756.

Entwistle V, O'Donnell M (2001). Evidence-based health care: what roles for patients? In: Edwards A, Elwyn G (eds) *Evidence-Based Patient Choice*. Oxford: Oxford University Press, 34–49.

Giddens A (1991). *Modernity and Self Identity: Self and Society in the Late Modern Age*. Cambridge: Polity.

Greenhalgh T (2001). Narrative and patient choice. In: Edwards A, Elwyn G (eds) *Evidence-Based Patient Choice*. Oxford: Oxford University Press.

Hall D (1980). Prescribing as social exchange. In: Mapes R (ed.) *Prescribing Practice and Drug Usage*. London: Croom Helm.

Hardey M (1999). Doctor in the house: the Internet as a source of lay health knowledge and the challenge to expertise. *Sociol Health Illness* 21: 820–835.

Helman C G (1978). "Feed a cold, starve a fever": folk models of infection in an English suburban community, and their relation to medical treatment. *Culture, Med Psychiatry* 2: 107–137.

Holman H, Lorig K (2000). Patients as partners in managing chronic disease. *BMJ* 320: 526–527.

Howie J G R, Heaney D J, Maxwell M, Walker J J (1998). A comparison of a patient enablement instrument (PEI) against two established satisfaction scales as an outcome measure of primary care consultations. *Fam Pract* 15: 165–171.

Katon W, Kleinman A (1981). Doctor–patient negotiation and other social science strategies in patient care. In: Eisenbergh L, Kleinman A (eds) *The Relevance of Social Science in Medicine*. London: D. Reidel, 253–279.

Makoul G, Arntson P, Schofield T P (1995). Health promotion in primary care: physician–patient communication and decision making about prescription medications. *Soc Sci Med* 41: 1241–1254.

Mechanic D (1992). Health and illness behavior and patient–practitioner relationships. *Soc Sci Med* 34: 1345–1350.

Mishler E G (1984). *The Discourse of Medicine. Dialectics of Medical Interviews*. New Jersey: Ablex.

Morgan M (1996). Perceptions and use of anti-hypertensive drugs among cultural groups. In: Williams S J, Calnan M (eds) *Modern Medicines: Lay Perspectives and Experiences*. London: UCL Press, 95–116.

Nettleton S (1995). *The Sociology of Health and Illness*. Cambridge: Polity.

NHS Executive (1996). *Patient Partnership: Building a Collaborative Strategy*. Leeds: NHS Executive.

Ong L M, de Haes J C, Hoos A M, Lammes F B (1995). Doctor–patient communication: a review of the literature. *Soc Sci Med* 40: 903–918.

Pollock K (2001). 'I've not asked him, you see and he's not said': understanding lay explanatory models of illness is a prerequisite for concordance consultations. *Int J Pharm Pract* 9: 105–117.

Sackett D L, Snow J C (1979). The magnitude of compliance and non-compliance. In: Haynes R B, Taylor W D, Sackett D L (eds) *Compliance in Health Care*, pp. 11–22. London: Johns Hopkins University Press.

Scambler G, Britten N (2001). System, lifeworld and doctor–patient interaction: issues of trust in a changing world. In: Scambler G (ed.) *Habermas, Critical Theory and Health*. London: Routledge.

Silverman D (1987). Communication and Medical Practice: Social Relations in the Clinic. London: Sage.

Smith R (2001). One Bristol, but there could have been many. *BMJ* 323: 179–180.

Stevenson F A, Wallace G, Rivers P, Gerrett D (1999). 'It's the best of two evils': a study of patients' perceived information needs about oral steroids for asthma. *Health Expectations* 2: 185–194.

Stevenson F A, Barry C A, Britten N *et al*. (2000). Doctor–patient communication about drugs: the evidence for shared decision making. *Soc Sci Med* 50: 829–840.

Stewart M A (1995). Effective physician–patient communication and health outcomes: a review. *Can Med Assoc J* 152: 1423–1433.

Stewart M, Brown J B (2001). Patient-centredness in medicine. In: Edwards A, Elwyn G (eds) *Evidence-Based Patient Choice*. Oxford: Oxford University Press.

Stewart M, Brown J B, Weston W W *et al*. (1995). *Patient-Centered Medicine – Transforming the Clinical Method*. London: Sage.

Stimson G, Webb B (1975). *Going to see the Doctor: The Consultation Process in General Practice*. London: Routledge & Kegan Paul.

Strong P M (1979). Sociological imperialism and the profession of medicine. A critical examination of the thesis of medical imperialism. *Soc Sci Med* 13: 199–215.

Tuckett D, Boulton M, Olson C, Williams A (1985). *Meetings Between Experts. An Approach to Sharing Ideas in Medical Consultations.* London: Tavistock.

Williams G H, Wood P H (1986). Common-sense beliefs about illness: a mediating role for the doctor. *Lancet* 2: 1435–1437.

4

The prescriber's perspective

Jon Dowell

Introduction

This chapter will consider how the shift towards concordance is affecting the clinicians who prescribe and the prescribing component of the consultation. It is deliberately aimed at all current as well as potential future prescribers because professional roles are changing rapidly and the underlying issues are generally the same. The term 'clinician' is, therefore, used throughout to represent doctor, dentist, pharmacist or nurse who may be in the position of discussing the use of or authorising supply of medicines. Although the vast majority of decisions about treatment are currently made between doctor and patient, there is little doubt that, at least in the UK, other professions will be expected to take increasing responsibility in this area. Although this may create some extra complications in terms of interprofessional issues, the clinician–patient interaction will be comparable. It is also likely that existing research on the prescribing process, which has mostly studied doctor–patient interactions, can be transferred to other professionals when they are involved in this previously 'medical' component of care. Although it will become increasingly important for research to be multidisciplinary, it would be foolish to ignore over 30 years of work studying medical encounters. This chapter invites readers to consider the relevance of existing quantitative and qualitative data to their own context. The application of concordance in practice is then considered under the headings of:

- how concordance affects the clinical decision-making process
- its impact on communication
- who wants concordance and when?
- how practitioners can be helped to adopt concordance

It closes with a discussion about controversial issues and potential solutions or the need for further study.

What do we know about the prescribing process and medication use?

There is a vast array of literature that is relevant to the content and process of decision-making about prescribed treatment. This section therefore does not claim to be a systematic review. Indeed, one problem is the quality of the studies available due to the complexity of researching interventions to change behaviours. This point is emphasised in the most rigorous systematic reviews to date (Haynes *et al.*, 1996; Ebrahim, 1998). The authors suggest seven criteria for intervention trials in this area, including studies where the placebo group also receives an alternative form of 'attention' and interventions that are applicable in clinical practice (e.g. not provided by research staff). However they found no studies that fulfilled these. The difficulties of conducting robust trials of new consultation approaches are huge and some equal insights are now emerging from qualitative studies that explore and explain the processes involved.

From the clinician's perspective it is important to consider the ways in which medicines are used because there is considerable evidence that 'compliant' patients have favourable medical outcomes. For instance, this has been reported in tuberculosis (Fox, 1983a, 1983b), hypertension (Meyer *et al.*, 1985; McKenney *et al.*, 1992), diabetes (Morris *et al.*, 1997) and myocardial infarction prevention (Franks *et al.*, 1992). Indeed, the act of complying may itself be beneficial and at least six randomised controlled trials have reported improved hard outcomes amongst patients who adhered to placebo regimens (Horwitz and Horwitz, 1993). One high-quality trial evaluating the efficacy of lipid-lowering drugs on mortality found an equal drop in mortality amongst those who complied with clofibrate and placebo (The Coronary Drug Project Research Group, 1980). So, being an individual who complies with treatment, even a placebo treatment, as designed confers benefit, though how much is due to pharmacological and how much to psychological effects is less clear.

It is also important to consider the impact of the consultation as a number of trials have now been conducted that assess the effect of altered communication with patients, for instance explicit involvement in decision-making. Stewart (1995) systematically reviewed 21 studies that compared aspects of doctor–patient communication and health outcome. These covered a wide range of conditions, outcomes and interventions, including assessment of doctor and patient statement types; extended discussion; patient-centred physician training; patient education; shared decision-making and consultation style. Overall, 16 of the 21 studies found significant positive health improvements suggesting that:

1. History-taking that included patient feelings, support and empathy improved symptom resolution, functional status and disease control (e.g. blood pressure).
2. Discussion of management plans improved emotional state, function, symptoms and disease control (e.g. glycosylated haemoglobin and blood pressure).

Another, less robust but interesting study by Thomas (1987) compared a 'positive' ('confident' doctor with clear assurances about recovery) with an 'ambivalent' (lack of certainty expressed) consultation style in managing minor illnesses. He found 64% of patients receiving a 'positive' approach recovered compared to 39% in the 'ambivalent' group, which was a greater effect than the prescription of a placebo treatment. Hence, there is reasonable evidence that enhanced doctor–patient communication can improve health outcomes. It is clear that, whatever changes may be introduced in patient information, the dispensing process or drug formulation, addressing the content and format of consultations is of key importance in improving outcomes (Blenkinsopp et al., 1997; Coulter et al., 1999). It is less clear how this can be implemented to maximal effect.

Decision-making

In Chapter 2 the emerging decision-making models and skills were outlined, and discussed from the patient's perspective in Chapter 3. Clinicians have the task of making these work in practice. It is clear that this has not been the case in the past and this component of the interaction has been termed the 'forgotten second half' of the consultation (Elwyn et al., 1999). Fortunately the shift towards a more patient-centred style of diagnostic encounter puts clinicians in a good position to include, explore and value the patient's perspective on treatment options much as they increasingly consider their views of the illness. Although the original writings on the patient-centred clinical method included the setting of goals and roles during a stage entitled 'mutual decision', this component was not heavily emphasised. In recent years authors such as Towle, Godolphin, Edwards, Elwyn, Silverman and Kurtz (Silverman et al., 1998; Towle and Godolphin, 1999; Edwards and Elwyn, 2002) have all presented essentially similar suggestions for achieving more shared decisions. The concordance initiative has provided the impetus or challenge to existing practice that should motivate clinicians to adopt these approaches. Unfortunately, motivation is required because it necessitates at least as much of a shift in attitude as skills. Firstly, clinicians have to adjust to the emergence of patient choice or power. Secondly, they must recognise the failure of the paternalistic style to achieve satisfactory patterns of treatment use. Finally, they are being asked to make a leap of faith and hope that, on balance, trusting patients to make informed decisions about their health will be beneficial, or at least no worse than the existing situation. For it must be acknowledged that the evidence for improved clinical outcomes is still being gathered (Stewart, 1995; Mead and Bower, 2002).

There is, of course, a wide range of circumstances that need considering. These range from finely balanced decisions between reasonable options at one level, to more challenging extremes when patients may choose a route with which the clinician strongly disagrees. Examples might include preference for laparoscopic compared to open surgery, declining treatment that could be life-saving or demanding a drug for which there is no evidence of benefit. Most clinicians would happily offer choice when the options were finely balanced, but might also present information in a leading way when they had firm views. The option of no treatment or other 'clinically inferior' options may often not even be mentioned. This situation is not helped by the increasing expectation that treatment must be predetermined by 'evidence-based' guidelines. This could become a substantial deterrent to concordance. Standard algorithms rarely include an allowance for patients' values and opinions. Computer-based decision aids may offer the potential to do so and recent studies have explored the use of such tools (Montgomery *et al.*, 2003). Finally, one special circumstance merits consideration. Patients often do not use medicines or behave as their clinicians have advised and can be seen as 'non-compliant'. Some will be deliberately exercising their right to make their own choices but this can be difficult to raise because patients are often thought to mislead in these circumstances (Tashkin *et al.*, 1991). They may feel intimidated or foolish and the clinician may feel disappointed or inadequate. However, there is evidence that a positive, sensitive approach that seeks discussion leading to concordance, and not compliance, can prove fruitful (Dowell *et al.*, 2002). The crux of concordance emerges when clinicians are asked to support patients who elect, knowingly, to choose or use a treatment contrary to best practice. Is supporting what could be seen as suboptimal treatment actually best practice (Montgomery and Fahey, 2001)?

Communication

There is a wealth of information revealing weaknesses in clinical communication with patients in the UK and many other countries. This applies across all specialties and professional groups and increasingly specific training is being introduced for undergraduates and postgraduates.

The value of improved, more patient-centred communication, as measured by improved clinical outcomes, has been shown by Stewart (1995) but there remains plenty of room for debate about which components are most important and how it leads to improved outcomes. Some of the most striking data has been provided by Greenfield and Kaplan *et al.* They tested 20 minutes of training for patients prior to consultations for diabetics ($n = 59$), hypertensives ($n = 105$) and peptic ulcer sufferers ($n = 45$) (Greenfield *et al.*, 1985, 1988; Kaplan *et al.*, 1989). These trials demonstrated clear and consistent changes within consultations that produced both functional and physiological improvements using sound design and including an attention control. It seems, therefore, that either party may generate effective change within doctor–patient interactions.

Overall these studies suggest that patients who are more actively involved in explaining their symptoms, understanding their illness or in discussing treatment tend to be more satisfied and have improved outcomes. However, it must be recognised that research in this area is extremely difficult and requires complex methods to allow for the effects of patient and physician self-selection, clustering and other effects. (Clustering effects complicate studies that evaluate training interventions as clinicians usually then apply their skills to a group of patients. The study sample must allow for the number of clinicians as well as the number of patients in case other clinician characteristics introduce confounding variation.) There have also been studies of patient-centred care that have shown little impact and more detailed studies are required (Kinmonth *et al.*, 1998; Mead and Bower, 2002).

Improved patient-centred consulting, which may improve diagnosis and satisfaction, is not the same as achieving shared decisions about treatment. For this to be achieved, close attention has to be paid to both the manner and process, as outlined above. Increasingly, studies are scrutinising the detail of the language and intonation used with techniques such as discourse analysis. One recent study assessed surgeons' communication style and compared this to their record of litigation claims (Ambady *et al.*, 2002). The researchers found briefly trained medical students could distinguish a clinician's propensity to be sued from hearing 20 seconds of consultation. So there is clearly much work to be done on the detail of approaching shared decisions.

Another difficulty in doctor–patient communication is the consistent finding that patients' accounts of medicine use overestimate actual use. This apparently inevitable finding (Stone *et al.*, 2002) unfortunately influences clinicians' views of all patients, which is unfair and unhelpful. The concordance initiative offers one potential escape from this. Studies commonly compare patient self-report of the average amounts of treatment taken with a more reliable measure. Where a discrepancy is identified, this suggests that many, if not most, patients might be considered liars. However, a patient's openness or honesty may vary in the context of a research study or a clinical encounter where the aim is to provide help. This is suggested by one study assessing compliance with digoxin using preconsultation interviews compared to biochemical assessments (Fletcher *et al.*, 1979). These investigators were able to gather accounts of non-compliance from 21 of the 24 who were not taking their digoxin according to serum measurements, suggesting that the precise way these topics are approached influences the outcome greatly. Hence, in an appropriately non-judgemental climate, in a therapeutic relationship where the patient feels cared for, not vulnerable or suspected, it should be possible to engender open discussion about treatment use, even with a majority of patients who do not use treatment 'as prescribed'. This may require not only refined consultation skills but also a perceptible change in professional attitudes so that patients feel themselves to be partners in their care and legitimately able to act according to their preferences without implied criticism. A genuine shift in culture is required to prevent mixed messages being given by different individuals and subsequent confusion. This may also require a change in record-keeping or even prescribing that conveys more than a basic instruction and includes a summary of the patient's views. Although some would argue this is done already, clearly it is not done enough.

Everyone is aware of the time pressures within the NHS and it is clear that patients, as well as clinicians, are acutely aware of the available time and limit themselves appropriately (Cromarty, 1996). However, we would not expect a surgeon to attempt an operation in inadequate time as that would clearly lead to failure or complications. Perhaps, as we increasingly understand the role of different components of the consultation, it is time to argue for moving beyond the average 9.9 minutes in the UK (Cape, 2002). Not all trials of increased consultation length have shown improved patient outcomes but if it can be shown that additional time is required to achieve concordance, and that this improves patient care, we must be prepared to argue the case for sufficient time to do the job properly.

Implications for practice

In practical terms prescribers need to consider when a concordant style is, or is not, appropriate, how to modify their own consulting style to offer it, and how to manage controversial issues such as variance with colleagues, related communication and clinical record-keeping. These are each considered here.

Who wants concordance?

Unfortunately there is conflicting evidence about what style of interaction patients want. In 1987 Thomas found that a GP's apparent confidence and directive style had a greater impact on recovery from non-specific minor infections than the prescription of a placebo tablet (Thomas, 1987, 1994). All doctors will have encountered colleagues who believe it is always best to appear confident and decisive in their advice, even when they are aware there are alternative options that they have elected not to mention, perhaps for fear of appearing less competent. There is also evidence that most patients prefer doctors to dress in an authoritative, somewhat traditional formal way, perhaps to reinforce the expected authority of the role (McKinstry and Wang, 1991).

There is, therefore, conflict between studies showing that patient involvement is beneficial, and a common belief supported by some evidence that providing decisive guidance has merits. The solution is surely to recognise that patients vary and that their needs will vary depending on the nature of their problem and situation. At times of acute, critical illness, even the most involved, articulate, intellectual individual is unlikely to want to discuss the options in detail. For instance, those suffering a suspected myocardial infarction may feel best cared for by a clinician who gives clear direction about the need for initiating therapy with aspirin and thrombolysis. They are vulnerable, have little autonomy and are likely to feel relieved if they can simply place trust in their carers. However, the same individual may be eager to be well informed and involved in decisions about subsequent long-term treatments such as antihypertensive agents, anticoagulants or lipid-lowering therapy. Indeed, they may be unlikely simply to accept advice or such treatments if they do not feel their views have been considered. So not only is there a variety of what might be called types of patients, but patients may also change preferences depending on their situation. The challenge for clinicians, then, is to be able to offer a range of styles of decision-making and be able to assess which is most appropriate during any one consultation.

Before going on to consider how clinicians can assess their patients' preferred role in this process it is important to consider that each party's role does not start from scratch, even in a first consultation about a new condition.

Powerful traditions have evolved that now govern expected and normally acceptable roles within medical encounters. These are extremely useful, as they enable the exchange of intimate information and physical examinations to be performed. However, there is also a substantive imbalance in power that still underlies most interactions. This has been described in the sociological literature and is undoubtedly crucial to understanding the philosophical shift that is represented by 'from compliance to concordance'. This is so deeply ingrained that clinical language continues to presume upon it greatly. For instance, the words 'prescribe', 'comply' or even 'adhere' all assume medical authority over a more passive recipient. This paternalistic presumption, although generally well intentioned, must be recognised for what it is and the effects that it has. One effect is to make it difficult for many patients to discuss openly the way they use or wish to use treatment for fear of courting criticism, jeopardising the clinical relationship or perhaps implying criticism in the prescriber. Consequently, clinicians who commence consultations with a paternalistic or traditional style, even if they are genuinely willing and able to change their style, will have begun by reinforcing the prevailing model of interaction, made their patients less likely to discuss their situation openly and made the task of changing style more difficult. Achieving concordance, therefore, requires a shift towards a patient-centred approach from the outset, because this will be instrumental in setting the tone of the encounter and encouraging patients – indeed empowering them – to be open about their views and planned or actual behaviour. Token statements such as: 'I know many people find taking their tablets every day difficult' before enquiring 'so do you often miss yours?' is rarely sufficient to overcome the powerful underlying expectations. However, the prevailing model of doctor–patient interaction is gradually becoming more patient-centred and will inevitably continue to so so. This need not be seen as a threat, rather an opportunity to develop a more constructive partnership that devolves more responsibility to the individual. It is also worth reflecting for a moment on the 'patient as consumer' transition. For consumers rarely demand things they do not know of. Patients, therefore, cannot be expected or relied upon to seek, let alone demand, a style of inter-action in which they are actively involved in decisions because they may never have experienced it. Perhaps many 'don't know what they are missing'?

The question has therefore become 'when is concordance not appropriate and how can clinicians find out?' not 'who wants concord-ance?' One important caveat is that we are currently focused on the vast majority of patients who are legally competent to manage their health-care decisions (or have a competent guardian/parent) and that the situ-ation is not complicated by a risk to others. For instance, certain infectious diseases, mental illnesses or drug abuse should be considered separately. Although seeking concordance and willing therapeutic par-ticipation may still be desirable, there are different legal responsibilities on clinicians that may preclude them from allowing such patients to make certain decisions.

Having clarified those rare occasions when concordance is not appropriate for legal and ethical reasons, we come to the key issue. How can clinicians establish with patients what role they seek to play in deciding about treatment? Undoubtedly this remains an inexact process and it must always rely heavily on the subtleties of interpersonal communication (Silverman *et al.*, 1998; Stewart *et al.*, 2003). It is none the less appropriate to consider the steps that might be required and the reasoning behind them.

We have established there is a sound reason for starting from the presumption that patients will usually be helped more by interactions in which, should they wish, they feel able to become involved in decision-making. This is to offset the traditional culture of paternalism in the medical encounter and open the door to patient participation. In addi-tion, those patients who are using their treatments in a 'non-compliant' fashion are already indicating, in a very pragmatic way, their need to be involved in a discussion about their views. Of course, creating an ambience that values patients' views, and explicitly including them in decisions will also make it easier for them to report their treatment use openly. As we know, most 'non-compliance' is not currently reported accurately, so anything that makes it easier for patients to disclose 'non-compliance' should be welcomed and seen as one way of establishing a clear need to revisit treatment decisions with that patient. So a primary component of concordant consultations is beginning to take shape. *The clinician will have an attitude that values patients' views and accepts their autonomy.* S/he will acknowledge the implicit impact of medical power and, therefore, recognise the need to establish more balanced encounters from the outset in order to help empower patients. S/he will note obvious signs of patients becoming involved in decisions about their treatment and recognise 'non-compliance' as one such sign.

But still we have not addressed the skills or techniques that might be useful for establishing who does or does not want to participate openly in treatment decisions. This is deliberate because these techniques are meaningless if patients do not perceive a genuine willingness to let them take responsibility and make their own decisions. This does not imply a lack of support, such as would occur if patients were offered information and left to sort it out for themselves, or the absence of any opinion about the most appropriate actions from the clinician. It does imply a willingness to support patients in making the best choices for them as individuals. On many occasions this will, at least initially, be the option favoured by the clinician but by implication it beholds the clinician to ensure the patient is aware there are alternatives, and to present these fairly. Not everyone will show interest in hearing about the alternatives, but if they do, they need information in an unbiased form. It does not value patients' autonomy to present, or 'frame', the information in a way that makes it difficult for them to choose other options. Statements such as: 'Would it help if I suggested what I think might be best and explain why?' can allow clinicians to assess how much the patient values their opinion or holds his or her own views. Responses such as: (1) 'You just tell me what to do, doctor, you're the boss'; (2) 'Yes, tell me what you would do'; (3) 'Well, I would like to know more about ...'; (4) 'I think I would like ...' are clear indications of the approach the patient is seeking from the clinician.

The tone of the response conveys a clear message about the patient's desire for involvement without necessarily explicitly asking. Those asking for guidance can be given it with a simple confirmatory check – 'How does that sound?' or perhaps, 'Would you like me to describe the alternatives or is that enough for now?' for those a little less keen on being directed.

An alternative commonly outlined in the literature on shared decision making is to assess formally what is termed the role preference.

These phrases can work well, especially to clarify the situation if it is unclear how a patient wishes to operate, or is conveying mixed messages. However, they can be awkward to introduce if used too early and can risk courting a defensive, traditional response of 'Well, you're the expert' if posed before the patient feels safe enough to assume some control. For those interested in developing their own approach further, then *Patient-Centered Medicine* (Stewart *et al.*, 2003) and *Skills for Communicating with Patients* (Silverman *et al.*, 1998) are recommended as useful texts. There is emerging evidence that training can improve clinicians' ability to involve patients in their decisions. So, in addition to a willingness to encourage patient autonomy, an awareness of power within medical interactions and an ability to foster a supportive relationship, we have now added some subtle communication skills. These are:

1. an ability to hear and respond to patients' cues about their preferred role
2. a method of confirming your interpretation and letting the patient back into the discussion if not
3. some phrases useful for exploring this issue if it is thought best to make it explicit

Again, however, it must be emphasised that these cannot work if the clinician does not believe it is right to give the patient the final choice.

One common scenario deserves special mention because it may require a more sophisticated approach and may particularly present to community pharmacists or nurses running chronic disease management clinics. That is when the record of prescriptions or dispensings indicates a patient cannot be complying (Beardon *et al.*, 1993; Morris *et al.*, 1997). This may present a challenging situation, especially if it is clear that clinical care is suboptimal, for instance poor blood pressure or diabetic control. It can be tempting in such circumstances to challenge patients with your knowledge in the hope that this will improve treatment use, but this could induce patients simply to request and collect future medicines but still not take them (Dowell and Hudson, 1997).

As described in Chapter 3, most patients have firm views about their medicines and often there is a need for discussion, review or at least some further information before they are likely to alter their behaviour. Any perceived pressure without an effort to understand their situation and reasoning is likely to provoke a feeling of resistance and may be counterproductive (Miller and Rollnick, 1991). It will also re-inforce the paternalistic model outlined earlier in this chapter and therefore reduce patients' willingness to be open about their treatment. When this situation is encountered it has proved more effective to focus initially on the desired clinical goal, or level of control sought (by the patient) as this is less emotive. Once an appropriate atmosphere has been created then, with care, treatment use can be explored (Dowell *et al.*, 2002).

Controversial issues

Concordance, as a way of practice, produces a number of controversial issues for clinicians. Some of these, such as establishing who wants it, how various professionals can be enabled to practise it and how to offer it, have already been discussed under implications for practice, above. Not all practitioners will find those issues of attitude and skills controversial, but many will. However, everyone should be aware of a number of potential problems with the practical application of concordance. These are variation in professional approach, assessing competence, communication between professionals and note-keeping, the value of clinical interventions/time spent seeking concordance and evidence of effect on outcome. Each is discussed briefly here.

Throughout this chapter it has been presumed that the clinician conferring with the patient has the authority to advise patients and when necessary support patients who choose to use or decline treatments in ways that counter what might be seen as best practice. This presents difficulty when there are clear guidelines on best practice, as has already been alluded to. This is likely to be a particular problem for non-medical clinicians working according to set protocols and changes in professional practice may be required to support this. The difficulties this creates for those working under more regulated conditions, particularly nurses and community pharmacists, needs to be recognised. Although many may already have developed a pragmatic approach and be working with patients using a concordant approach, problems may arise if there is not a clear understanding with the responsible clinician, commonly a doctor.

There are several scenarios. Let us consider a female hypertensive patient attending for review with a nurse. During the consultation it becomes apparent that she does not like or take her medication regularly and that her blood pressure is elevated. Using a concordant approach the nurse might explore what the patient felt about this and discover that this patient does not consider controlling her blood pressure is important. She may be aware of, or the nurse might clarify, the perceived benefit of reduced cardiovascular risks but this may not influence her views. She may even announce that she does not plan to attend for further review. What is the nurse to do? S/he could acknowledge it is the patient's choice and sanction her decision, which would conflict with most protocols. Does a nurse have the authority to do this? Alternatively, s/he could direct the patient to the doctor, which is in itself paternalistic but covers the nurse's responsibilities. Depending on his/her approach the doctor may be paternalistic and attempt to inform, cajole or frighten the patient into complying, which would deter any future revelations about treatment use to the nurse. Alternatively, the doctor might review the patient's knowledge and views and use a concordant approach to negotiate an acceptable course of action. The same dilemma could easily arise in a pharmacy and it is therefore important that the difficulty of working to protocols or regulations and attempting to achieve concordance is recognised. Whilst there remains wide variation in how different professions or indeed individual professionals respond to patients, there is a need for local discussion and clarity. Whether it is between consultant and house officer, GP and practice nurse or prescriber and dispensing pharmacist, this transition is likely to generate discrepancies and risks conveying mixed messages to patients. It would be helpful if researchers could identify workable solutions to this dilemma.

If patients are to make decisions that might affect their future health or, indeed, lifespan, they need to be competent. However, assessing this will not always be a simple matter. Difficult scenarios might include patients with learning disability, early dementia, teenagers or those with a parent or guardian whose limits of responsibility are being reached. The recently introduced incapacity legislation in the UK has put the responsibility for such assessments explicitly on to the prescriber but unfortunately offers very little guidance on exactly how this should be done or what criteria should be applied. Although the legal principle of patient autonomy is now well established, it is important for clinicians to have considered (and recorded) when such autonomy is appropriate. They must also explain any substantive risks and confirm that the risks have been understood. If this is done, and documented, prescribers can feel content that they have discharged their responsibilities adequately. The importance of having a clearly established practice for this process cannot be overemphasised, as clinicians cannot feel free to discuss all options openly unless they are happy to let patients choose one that would not be recommended. However, enhanced record-keeping and communication is required for clinicians to convey and record the discussions they have had with patients along with the roles, goals and actions that have been agreed in a legally robust way. Legal experts and the medical defence societies could help clarify acceptable standards for this process.

Is seeking concordance an effective use of time?

There is a major assumption underlying the concordance initiative that must be acknowledged and urgently researched before practice changes. Robust evidence of the impact of this process is needed. The concordance initiative developed from frustration with the failure of efforts to improve compliance and the increasing recognition that some patients not only seek to be, but also should be, active in choices about their treatment. The motivation of those involved was to try and understand why patients were not complying with treatment advice, and therefore not obtaining optimal benefit available from powerful, often expensive, modern drugs.

As a best-case scenario, engaging all patients in open discussion could convince everyone to choose an appropriate treatment with which they would then comply to the best of their ability. This would undoubtedly improve clinical management and be considered a success from the clinical perspective. An alternative scenario would involve many patients seeking more relaxed treatment goals or electing not to take treatment. They may be happy to have been involved and made their own treatment decisions but clinical outcomes would be worse. Clearly the likely outcome of adopting concordant practice on a wide scale lies somewhere in between. But where would it have to lie to be judged worthwhile?

This is an extremely vexing issue to research as it involves rating individual and perhaps societal values in addition to identifying worthwhile, sensitive clinical outcome markers and valid assessments of treatment used. If someone elected not to take treatment for hypertension, knowingly accepting increased risk and consequently had a stroke, how should that be judged? A success because their view was respected, a failure to convince the patient of risk, or irresponsible care? On a wider scale, how much training and professional time is it worth investing in a process that might be appreciated by many patients but could produce no net benefit in terms of reduced morbidity or mortality? Is there a simple ethical imperative to move practice in this direction, or do we require more robust evidence of some form of overall benefit first?

Of course the conundrum posed above is itself inappropriately simplistic, because practitioners are sensible and selective, and would tailor their time investment according to perceived need. For instance, recently I treated a young man who became rapidly short of breath and was diagnosed with two heart conditions – atrial fibrillation and cardiomyopathy. Diabetes mellitus was confirmed a few months later. He was shocked and unable to engage constructively with his hospital or primary care advisers. He failed to attend appointments and complied poorly with medication, including warfarin. He was clearly at a high risk of numerous unfortunate events. Investing some time in exploring this man's knowledge, beliefs and attitude towards his situation and his treatment options proved critical in re-engaging him in a constructive therapeutic relationship. The payback from investing time selectively in such patients will be far greater than in a study with a less focused intervention.

It can be argued that research studying the effects of using a concordant approach should, therefore, focus initially on those patients who stand most to gain, e.g. those who are known to have poor control of their condition and be using treatment suboptimally. If it is shown that seeking concordance benefits such patients, in the broadest sense, then further work is required in other groups. If studies recruit less highly selected groups of patients they risk missing the main benefit. Sampling non-compliant hypertensives identified from a practice record of prescriptions, for instance, risks focusing in a paternalistic way on compliance, irritating patients and producing no benefit in terms of patient involvement or clinical control. Studies training practitioners to share all treatment decisions more would need to pay greater attention to time costs and patient preferences. How the success of concordance is judged may depend greatly on the context of its application.

The way forward?

This section seeks to make positive suggestions for practice or research to help address the controversial issues raised above. There is no suggestion that these are the best, let alone the only alternatives, and this field is likely to develop and change rapidly. The following topics will be considered.

1. How to offer/select patients for concordance?
2. Can multiprofessional teams make concordance work?
3. How should clinical record-keeping and communication develop?
4. Assessing the value of concordance.

How to offer/select patients for concordance?

Applying a concordant approach in practice should perhaps be viewed as a spectrum of potential approaches, some of which many clinicians will already be practising. At its simplest, all patients can be offered the choice of becoming involved in treatment decisions. At this level, concordance is simply the continuation of the patient-centred approach into the 'closing half' of the consultation. It is already part of all consultation models based upon the patient-centred clinical method. Although not everyone will want a concordant style of interaction, and a formal inquiry into their decision-making preferences may be perceived as inappropriate, it is still possible to explore and include their values and wishes within the process. This is now a component of the Royal College of General Practitioner membership exam. However, it is difficult to change consultation style and many practitioners will require training to help them achieve this in a natural manner.

The ethos of concordance may also, and perhaps most effectively, be introduced when 'non-compliance' comes to light.

If all professionals could simply explore why patients use treatment as they do, using a genuinely inquiring manner without implying criticism, this would perform two important functions. Firstly, it would gradually help to destigmatise 'non-compliance' and help empower patients to be more open. Secondly, all professionals with existing active listening skills will naturally find themselves responding in a way that incorporates the patient's views. Such a change requires clinicians to accept that patients have the right to decide about treatment and avoid simply restating instructions. Some may need to change their approach and attitude substantively, which may only occur as part of a more general cultural shift in service provision.

Some patients are risking or suffering considerable harm due to their medication use, or non-use. Examples include symptomatic insulin use, irregular warfarin use and severe asthma attacks associated with scant use of effective preventive steroids. Commonly there are substantive issues blocking these patients' more appropriate use of treatment and often relationships with clinicians are poor as a direct consequence. Not surprisingly, such patients do not like to attend clinicians who they perceive lambast them for failing to comply. These patients' issues are unlikely to be substantively helped by a listening ear at the pharmacy counter, where irregular medication use can be detected from dispensing records, although pharmacists and their staff may be instrumental in re-engaging them with services. Exploring reasons and seeking resolution for these patients requires a more detailed and sophisticated approach, and possibly formal counselling. This role necessitates appropriate knowledge (of health behaviours and behaviour change), attitudes (towards patient autonomy) and skills (in patient-centred consulting, counselling and raising motivation). As an 'extended role', this might be ideal for clinicians from any discipline with a special interest and additional training. Non-medical practitioners may have the advantage of less entrenched consultation roles, as discussed earlier, and possibly less hierarchical professional–patient relationships. They would need to accept responsibility or have good working relationships with those who hold responsibilities for prescribing.

As an example, it would be ideal if patients whose anticoagulation was chaotic could be reviewed by a pharmacist able to explore their views about risks of a stroke, bleeding and use of warfarin as well as concomitant prescribing and diet. If, however, discussions concluded that this patient did not want to be on warfarin, a mechanism must be in place for recording and upholding this decision. It would be inefficient and counterproductive if anticoagulation was imposed when s/he next attended the GP or outpatient clinic.

Can multiprofessional teams make concordance work?

It is well recognised that different doctors, let alone different professionals, have varying styles of interaction with patients. We are used to working with this but concordance presents particular challenges. These already arise increasingly with the creation of practice-based pharmacists and nurse prescribing, and this will be exacerbated as pharmacist prescribing, including community pharmacists, is rolled out (Department of Health, 2003). How these usually tightly controlled, protocol-driven systems can accommodate concordance remains to be worked out. Qualitative studies will be required to explore how this may be done. It may well prove easy where there are effective relationships in place and clear direction and support are available from the local authority figure, be that consultant, GP or dentist. However, such authorised or supplementary prescribers will struggle to engage patients fully if they do not have adequate support. When they do, it is likely that some new record-keeping conventions will need to emerge as well as ways of setting boundaries to deviations from protocols to provide sufficient clarity and confidence.

One opportunity that this initiative offers is for individuals to develop special interests or skills managing more complex cases involving suboptimal treatment choices or use. Such patients are worthy of a greater time investment than many doctors can offer and a skilled nurse or pharmacist could play a valuable role. Clearly many specialist nurses and others are already heavily involved in encouraging and helping patients comply. With some additional skills, and appropriate collaboration from the prescriber, they would be ideally placed to conduct concordant consultations with patients whose psychological adjustments to ill health may be well known to them. However, they can only do so if their agreements with patients are understood, accepted and supported by the medical staff. There is, therefore, an opportunity for individuals to develop special skills in this topic and offer to 'accept referrals' from within their own clinical teams.

How should clinical record-keeping and communication develop?

There are two areas in which clinical records may need to develop to facilitate concordant practice. Firstly, a nomenclature for recording and presenting the diagnostic elements of the interaction must be established. Just as the relevance of various symptoms of depression or angina will be systematically recorded, maybe even rated on a standardised scale, it will help to record a more structured insight into medication use, for instance the information conveyed, relevant patient beliefs and values about their options and any practical issues that affect use. Once the 'compliance model' has been dropped and concordance accepted, it is a small step to accept that patients' motivation, understanding and attitude towards their medicines are key factors that need recording. This is required to help different clinicians avoid revisiting old territory many times and needs conveying to other involved parties within the normal correspondence. In this way decisions made by one clinician are conveyed to others and are not repeatedly challenged by others.

Secondly, the simplest legally robust form of recording an informed choice not to accept established advice or treatment needs to be determined so clinicians can feel confident that they are able genuinely to support patients' decisions without fear of litigation.

Assessing the value of concordance

There are many substantive methodological problems to be considered by those wishing to research the impact of concordance, and Chapter 7 addresses these more fully. However, it is useful for them also to be briefly summarised here:

1. What constitutes concordance? Is an assessment of the process or interaction to be used or the outcome? This can be divided further into the

level of agreement between the parties, as the word implies, or the extent to which the patient's views were accepted, an integral component of the definition.

2.   What types of interaction should be studied? Are routine encounters appropriate, in which changes in treatment use, let alone outcome, may be difficult to detect? Or are patients with particular problems in treatment of more interest? Likewise, should broadly applicable, simple and quick attempts to achieve concordance be studied or are more complex special appointments, perhaps with some type of subspecialist, more relevant? Or, as they are so different, should both be studied separately?

3.   As it is impossible to standardise the intervention, it might be best to test practitioner-training strategies and then study changes in clinical encounters and subsequent patient outcomes. This approach, however, requires sophisticated cluster randomised trials and defined objective outcome measures and therefore can be complex and expensive to run in practice.

4.   Whatever effect concordance has on consultations or patients' satisfaction with their involvement in the decisions made, it will be important to assess the impact on medication use and clinical outcomes. Interpreting these studies will be difficult as the process of engaging patients in a concordant approach may also alter their reporting of medication use. It might also be difficult to interpret clinical outcomes. If many patients elected, for instance, not to control their blood pressure tightly, then effective concordant consulting could lead to apparently worse clinical care. Is this failure?

Summary

This chapter has attempted to highlight some of the implications and practical issues for clinicians from any discipline eager to embrace the concordance ethos. The opportunity for medication use to be improved was reiterated and some of the literature illustrating the therapeutic potential of the consultation was introduced. Although it must be acknowledged that evidence for improved clinical outcomes resulting from involving patients is mixed and incomplete, there are considerable moral reasons for changing normal practice in this direction.

Although we cannot yet predict precisely how clinicians should consult to greatest effect during any one encounter, there is an emerging consensus on the key components of interactions that encourage patients to become involved if they wish. Combined with existing evidence that few clinicians currently use these techniques, there is clearly a substantial need for training.

There are a number of potentially difficult or controversial issues that arise from concordance. Some are practical: relearning consultation styles; avoiding interprofessional variation in approach; and enhanced record-keeping. These will evolve through experimentation and example. However, some fundamental issues remain for those appraising the value of concordance: how is its achievement to be measured and what outcomes will be valued? If patients' values or choices conflict with normal clinical priorities, will enabling patients be considered a success, especially if their health suffers in some way? That, after all, is the bottom-line decision with which every clinician needs to come to terms.

References

Ambady N, LaPlante D, Nguyen T *et al.* (2002). Surgeons' tone of voice: a clue to malpractice history. *Surgery* 132: 5–9.

Beardon P H G, McGilchrist M M, McKendrick A D *et al.* (1993). Primary non-compliance with prescribed medication in primary care. *BMJ* 307: 846–848.

Blenkinsopp A, Bond C, Britten N *et al.* (1997). *From Compliance to Concordance: Achieving Shared Goals in Medicine-taking.* London: Merck Sharp and Dohme, Royal Pharmaceutical Society of Great Britain.

Cape J (2002). Consultation length, patient-estimated consultation length and satisfaction with the consultation. *Br J Gen Pract* 52: 1004–1006.

Coulter A, Entwistle V A, Gilbert D (1999). Sharing decisions with patients: is the information good enough? *BMJ* 318: 318–322.

Cromarty J (1996). What do patients think about their consultations? A qualitative study. *Br J Gen Pract* 46: 525–528.

Department of Health (2003). *Supplementary Prescribing by Nurses and Pharmacists Within the NHS in England. A Guide for Implementation.* London: Department of Health.

Dowell J S, Hudson H (1997). A qualitative study of medication taking behaviour in primary care. *Family Pract* 14: 369–375.

Dowell J, Jones A, Snadden D (2002). Exploring medication use to seek concordance with 'non-adherent' patients: a qualitative study. *Br J Gen Pract* 52: 24–32.

Ebrahim S (1998). Detection, adherence and control of hypertension for the prevention of stroke: a systematic review. *Health Technol Assess* 2 (11): 1–78.

Edwards A, Elwyn G (2002). *Evidence-based Patient Choice, Inevitable or Impossible?* Oxford: Oxford University Press.

Elwyn G, Edwards A, Kinnersley P (1999). Shared decision-making in primary care: the neglected second half of the consultation. *Br J Gen Pract* 49: 477–482.

Fletcher S W, Pappius E M, Harper S J (1979). Measurement of medication in a clinical setting. Comparison of three methods in patients prescribed digoxin. *Arch Intern Med* 139: 635–638.

Fox W (1983a). Of patients and physicians: experience and lessons from tuberculosis – II. *BMJ* 287: 101–105.

Fox W (1983b). Of patients and physicians: experience and lessons from tuberculosis – I. *BMJ* 287: 33–35.

Franks P J, Sian M, Kenchington G F *et al.* (1992). Aspirin usage and its influence on femoro-popliteal vein graft patency. The femoro-popliteal bypass trial participants. *Eur J Vasc Surg* 6: 185–188.

Greenfield S, Kaplan S, Ware J (1985). Expanding patient involvement in care. *Ann Intern Med* 102: 520–528.

Greenfield S, Kaplan S, Ware J *et al.* (1988). Patients' participation in medical care: effects on blood sugar control and quality of life in diabetes. *J Gen Intern Med* 3: 448–457.

Haynes R B, McKibbon K A, Kanani R (1996). Systematic review of randomised trials of interventions to assist patients to follow prescriptions for medictions. *Lancet* 348: 383–386.

Horwitz R I, Horwitz S M (1993). Adherence to treatment and health outcomes. *Arch Intern Med* 153: 1863–1868.

Kaplan S, Greenfield S, Ware J (1989). Assessing the effects of physician–patient interactions on the outcomes of chronic disease. *Med Care* 27 (3): S110–S127.

Kinmonth A L, Woodcock A, Griffith S *et al.* (1998). Ramdomised controlled trial of patient centred care of diabetes in general practice: impact on current well-being and future disease risk. *BMJ* 317 (1167): 1202–1208.

McKenney J M, Munroe W P, Wright J T J (1992). Impact of an electronic medication aid on long-term blood pressure control. *J Clin Pharmacol* 32: 277–283.

McKinstry B, Wang J X (1991). Putting on the style: what patients think of the way their doctor dresses. *Br J Gen Pract* 41 (348): 270, 275–278.

Mead N, Bower P (2002). Patient-centred consultations and outcomes in primary care: a review of the literature. *Patient Educ Couns* 48: 51–61.

Meyer D, Leventhal H, Gutmann M (1985). Common-sense models of illness: the example of hypertension. *Health Psychol* 4 (2): 115–135.

Miller W R, Rollnick S (1991). *Motivational Interviewing*. New York: Guilford.

Montgomery A A, Fahey T (2001). How do patients' treatment preferences compare with those of clinicians? *Qual Health Care* 10 (suppl. I): i39–i43.

Montgomery A A, Fahey T, Peters T J (2003). A factorial randomised controlled trial of decision analysis and an information video plus leaflet for newly diagnosed hypertensive patients. *Br J Gen Pract* 53: 446–453.

Morris A D, Boyle D I R, McMahon A D *et al.* (1997). Adherence to insulin treatment, glycaemic control, and ketoacidosis in insulin-dependent diabetes mellitus. *Lancet* 350: 1505–1510.

Silverman J, Kurtz S M, Draper J (1998). *Skills for Communicating with Patients*. Oxford: Radcliffe Medical Press.

Stewart M A (1995). Effective physician–patient communication and health outcomes: a review. *Can Med Assoc J* 152 (9): 1423–1433.

Stewart M, Belle Brown J, Weston W W *et al.* (2003). *Patient-Centered Medicine. Transforming the Clinical Method*, 2nd edn. Abingdon, UK: Radcliffe Medical Press.

Stone A A, Shiffman S, Schwartz J E *et al.* (2002). Patient non-compliance with paper diaries. *BMJ* 324 (7347): 1193–1194.

Tashkin D P, Rand C, Nides M *et al.* (1991). A nebulizer chronolog to monitor compliance with inhaler use. *Am J Med* 91: 33S–36S.

The Coronary Drug Project Research Group (1980). Influence of adherence to treatment and response of cholesterol on mortality in the Coronary Drug Project. *N Engl J Med* 303: 1038–1041.

Thomas K B (1987). General practice consultations: is there any point in being positive? *BMJ* 294: 1200–1202.

Thomas K B (1994). The placebo in general practice. *Lancet* 344: 1066–1067.

Towle A, Godolphin W (1999). Framework for teaching and learning informed shared decision making. *BMJ* 319: 766–769.

5

Ongoing support – the postprescription phase

Alison Blenkinsopp

Introduction

The key to achieving concordance with treatment is for practitioners to establish a dialogue with the patient that elicits and addresses the patient's agenda. Patients need support in their medicine-taking, starting when a new treatment is prescribed, through monitoring of continued use, to review of effectiveness and appropriateness. This chapter will focus on treatment for chronic conditions in the primary care setting as this is where most medicine-taking occurs. It particularly addresses the postprescription phase and therefore is particularly relevant to all health and social care professionals.

At the initial supply of a new medicine the pharmacist can begin to identify patients' questions and information needs. During continued treatment, and resultant interaction with patients and their carers, all health professionals (particularly nurses and pharmacists) and social care staff have an opportunity to monitor medicines use and identify medicines-related problems. Medication review can address problems by modifying or stopping treatment where necessary. There can also be additional support in the form of information and advice, prompts and reminders, and compliance aids. This chapter draws on research findings to enable practitioners to increase their understanding of patient perspectives on treatment, match their consulting and support frameworks accordingly, and facilitate concordance. Recommendations for the future are made.

When a medicine is first prescribed

At this point a decision has been made about treatment and one or more medicines have been prescribed. That decision may or may not have been made with involvement of the patient, and the patient's intent to take the treatment may be unknown. Research has shown that 96% of patients have a particular agenda when they consult their GP (McKinley and Middleton, 1999). However, that agenda may not be expressed or elicited during the consultation and in their ground-breaking study of communication between patients and GPs, Barry and colleagues found that problem outcomes were often related to the treatment decision (Barry *et al.*, 2000). During interviews with patients after their consultation the researchers found that problems resulted:

> where a patient did not reveal that a prescription was not wanted, where side effects were not raised, or self-treatment was not mentioned (Barry *et al.*, 2000).

McKinley's study found that 69% of patients wanted an explanation of their condition by the doctor and 55% wanted a prescription (McKinley and Middleton, 1999). Where a prescription was not wanted or expected the patient may then have decided not to have the prescription dispensed ('primary non-compliance') (Schafheutle *et al.*, 2002). It cannot be assumed that just because patients present a prescription and collect the dispensed medicine that they intend to take the treatment as prescribed.

If the patient is a hospital inpatient the medicine will be administered, or at least supervised, by hospital staff and unless the patient refuses to take it, the doses will be given. However, the patient will subsequently be discharged and expected to continue the treatments advised by the hospital. The dispensing of discharge medicines is an opportunity for discussion but limited time may restrict the opportunity even to begin to address issues relevant to concordance. If the patient is attending an outpatient clinic, or has had a consultation with a doctor or nurse in the community, the prescription will be taken to a community pharmacy to be dispensed. There may be an opportunity at this point for the pharmacist to open a dialogue with the patient or carer.

There is evidence that health professionals have an agenda of information items that they believe need to be provided to the patient and that they have a view on relative priorities of different information items. However, research has also found a gap between these priorities, in this case, patients' and GPs' (Berry *et al.*, 1997) (Table 5.1).

Thus there is a need for health professionals to recognise that the patient may have different priorities for receiving information and take this into account. Research shows that patients ask few questions of pharmacists about their medicines and that most information is provided by the pharmacist without the patient asking for it (Blom *et al.*,

Table 5.1 Patients' and doctors' priorities for information about medicines

Information item	Patients' ranking	Doctors' ranking
Possible side-effects	1	10.5
What the medication does	2	10.5
Lifestyle changes	3	3
Detailed questions about taking the medication	4	2
What is the medicine (drug type; active ingredient)	5	15
Interaction with medicine prescribed for long-term use	6	1
What to do if symptoms change or don't change	7	10.5
Probability medication will be effective	8	14
Any alternatives to the medicine	9	16
Is it known to be effective?	10	13

Reproduced with permission from Berry *et al.* (1997). (*Psychology and Health* website available at www.tandf.co.uk.)

1998). In another study the question most patients (60%) most wanted to ask the pharmacist when collecting a new prescription was about side-effects (Chewning and Schommer, 1996). Patients in the same study were asked what stopped them from asking the pharmacist questions. Pharmacy barriers were cited by 18% (being handed the prescription by an assistant; the pharmacist being perceived as rude or abrupt; and inadequate privacy). A lack of awareness of what questions could or should be asked was cited by 20% of patients. Fear or embarrassment was cited by 22% of patients (Chewning and Schommer, 1996). These findings suggest that community pharmacists might want to consider:

1. displaying a notice to tell patients that their questions about medicines will be welcomed
2. asking patients directly what questions they have about their medicines
3. checking with the patient that the information they are giving is wanted

Support from the pharmacist

Pharmacists have a particular opportunity to support patients when medicines are first prescribed. International research indicates that community pharmacists spend 5.8–7.2% of their working time on health-related talk with their customers (Savage, 1999). The way in which that time is spent, the extent to which the discussion is pharma-cist- or patient-initiated and how it maps against patients' needs have not been well explored in research. A UK study of interactions between elderly people and community pharmacists found that pharmacists provided verbal information to 12.5% of patients about their pre-scribed medicines (Livingstone, 1996). Most of the information was about aspects of the dosage regimen and the average time spent in giv-ing the information was 71 seconds. Another UK study found that an 'average' patient with a prescription might expect to receive between 30 seconds and 1 minute of advice (Savage, 1997). The basis on which pharmacists selected patients for information-giving is unclear. However, research shows that patients receiving repeat prescriptions are less likely to receive advice than those presenting a first-time pre-scription (Livingstone et al., 1996; Savage, 1997).

Thus community pharmacists give a high priority to first-time pre-scriptions for medicines. In depression, for example, studies in the UK, Canada and the USA have shown that community pharmacists provide information for many patients when an antidepressant is first dispensed (Gardner et al., 2001, Bultman and Svarstad, 2002; Landers et al., 2002). A Canadian study found that between one-half and two-thirds of patients recalled their pharmacist inquiring about some or all of: past use of the antidepressant; discussing the written information pro-vided; mentioning how long it would take the treatment to work; and side-effects (Gardner et al., 2001). Areas discussed less frequently were the purpose of the antidepressant, target symptoms, usual duration of therapy and risk of relapse with premature discontinuation. The find-ings from our study of UK community pharmacists indicated that they actively provided information at the first point of dispensing an anti-depressant (Landers et al., 2002). Our ongoing research indicates that community pharmacists also see the dispensing of a new prescription for a lipid-regulating medicine as a time when key information should be provided about, for example, the timing of the dose (Chatterton et al., 2004).

Thus many pharmacists are already in the habit of discussing some aspects of prescribed medicines usage with the patient, particu-larly when the prescription is presented for the first time. Patients also have a thirst for more information, which is currently not universally met. It would seem that there could already be a foundation on which to build discussions to support concordance in the community phar-macy.

Monitoring of continued treatment

All health and social care professionals can contribute to treatment monitoring with referral of the patient to the appropriate colleague if problems are identified. In addition to patients' visits to the surgery or pharmacy, home visits offer an opportunity to discuss medication in the patient's own setting. Social services assessments can contribute to medication monitoring. In England, for example, the Single Assessment Process includes a brief set of basic questions about medicines to provide a screening function. It is also an opportunity to identify patients with more complex needs for onward referral to pharmacist or doctor.

Key questions in medication monitoring

A recent systematic review has considered the evidence about communication between health professionals and patients about medicine-taking (Cox *et al.*, 2004). Many patients have unanswered questions about their medicines and are reluctant to raise these questions. The results of the review suggest that health professionals need to respond by taking a more proactive role in asking patients questions about their medicine-taking.

Health professionals can consider asking five basic questions for use in treatment monitoring, with further action based on the patient's answers.

1. Is the patient taking/using the medicine?
2. Does the patient have any side-effects?
3. Are any monitoring tests being done regularly?
4. Does the patient feel s/he is benefiting from the medicine?
5. Does the patient need any help with the medicine?

These questions are considered in detail below.

Is the patient taking/using the medicine?

It is estimated that 50% of prescribed medicines are not taken or used as intended (Royal Pharmaceutical Society of Great Britain, 1997). Research has found that the extent to which patients follow instructions for prescribed medicines varies according to the condition being treated, as Table 5.2 shows.

However, research also shows that health professionals' estimates of patients' compliance are inaccurate. Although patients' self-reports have been criticised as a method for measuring compliance, carefully

Table 5.2   Rates of non-compliance by disease state

Condition	Rate of non-compliance
Contraception	8
Asthma	20
Epilepsy	30–50
Hypertension	40
Diabetes	40–50
Arthritis	55–71

Reproduced with permission from Berg *et al.* (1993).

worded questions enable patients to talk about medicines use without fearing the disapproval of the health professional. Studies of patients on chronic medication show that 20–30% express issues about adhering to their treatment (Montbriand, 2000; Sleath *et al.,* 2000). Patients' reasons for stopping medication or using it differently than prescribed were found in a USA study to be: not understanding the diagnosis; having unpleasant reactions; and costs of medicines (Montbriand, 2000).

By increasing their understanding of patients' ideas and beliefs about medicines, practitioners can establish a dialogue with patients about their medication. Patients' decisions about whether and how to take a medicine are complex and patients balance perceived positive and negative aspects of the medicine, making their own risk–benefit assessment (Benson and Britten, 2002). In the Benson and Britten study 29 of 38 patients with hypertension stated some reservations about taking their antihypertensive medication but at the same time they all also held positive perceptions about their treatment. Two-thirds of these 29 patients described balancing the positive and negative. The researchers developed a taxonomy of patients' perceptions about medication and this is reproduced in Box 5.1.

Practitioners can use this taxonomy to explore the patient's perspective. Although it was developed from research on antihypertensive medication, there is much of relevance and value to other chronic conditions.

Does the patient have any side-effects?

Asking patients whether they think they are experiencing any side-effects is an important part of monitoring treatment. Sometimes a side-effect may be mild; others may be more severe and require referral

Box 5.1 Patients' reservations about medicines and reasons to take antihypertensive drugs

Patients' reservations about medicines

Patients' reservations about drugs generally

- Drugs are best avoided
- Drugs are unnatural or unsafe
- Drugs are perceived adversely because of previous experience
- Drugs are signifiers of ill health
- Patient brought up to avoid drugs
- Doctors prescribe drugs too readily

Reservations about antihypertensive drugs specifically

- Desire to discontinue using antihypertensives
- Preference for an alternative to drugs
- Patient questioned continued necessity
- Possible long-term or hidden risks

Patients' reasons to take antihypertensive drugs

Positive experiences with doctors

- Advice from doctors
- Trust in doctors
- Improved blood pressure readings

Perceived benefits of medication

- Achieving a good outcome
- Feeling better
- Gaining peace of mind

Pragmatic considerations

- Absence of a practical alternative to drugs
- Absence of symptoms to guide medicine use
- Drug use overshadowed by some other consideration

Reproduced with permission from Benson and Britten (2002).

back to the prescriber. Additionally, side-effects perceived to be mild to the professional may be intolerable to the patient, to the extent that they compromise further medicine-taking.

The majority of side-effects brought to the attention of doctors and pharmacists were identified by patients (Houghton *et al.*, 1999). However, research shows that health professionals tend to believe that patients are likely to attribute new symptoms wrongly as the adverse effects of treatment (Hughes *et al.*, 2002) and that if patients are given more information about side-effects they are more likely to report experiencing them. In their study of 158 practice nurses, Lip and Beevers found that only 23% said they would tell a patient about side-effects without being asked (Lip and Beevers, 1996, 1997). More recent legislation requires that all dispensed medicines are supplied with a copy of the manufacturer's patient information leaflet (PIL) which has to include information about side-effects.

Are any monitoring tests being done regularly?

Another important aspect of maintaining patient safety is checking whether monitoring tests are being regularly conducted where these are required. A list of relevant medicines can be found at www.medicines-partnership.org. Not only is it important to check that tests are being done, but also that results have been reviewed and action taken if needed. Initiatives such as the National Kidney Federation's Know Your Numbers card inform patients about the reason why tests are important and what the results mean. This model could be transferred to other conditions. There may also be a case to involve patients in this process, and make them responsible at least in part for requesting the monitoring using an *aide-mémoire* like an appointment card.

Does the patient feel s/he is benefiting from the medicine?

Patients' beliefs about whether the medicine is benefiting them are central to discussions about concordance. Patients who are taking a medicine for a symptomatic condition will be able to measure the effect of the treatment. Those who are taking a medicine for an asymptomatic treatment may not have any such measure. Where the treatment is preventive, for example, in hypertension or hyperlipidaemia, levels are measured by a health professional. However, the patient may not always have been given (or may not have remembered) the explanation about why continued treatment is still needed. Even in a condition such as asthma, where a patient may have symptoms, there may be reluctance to use inhaled steroids continually and there is evidence that they are widely underused. Our research with patients with asthma found that some perceive their asthma as adequately controlled, even when a quality-of-life questionnaire demonstrated considerable symptom levels.

Thus asking the patient's view on benefit from the medicine can help to open up a discussion about how the patient feels about using the medicine. It is here that any misunderstandings can be talked through.

Does the patient need any help with the medicine?

Simply asking patients if they need any help can open a dialogue about what sorts of problems are being experienced and what further support might be needed.

Who is responsible for monitoring?

Although all health professionals can play a part in monitoring, there is some uncertainty about who is responsible for ensuring it is done. Nurses and pharmacists may perceive that monitoring is the responsibility of the prescriber. In their work with community mental health nurses, for example, Jordan and colleagues found that, although the nurses recognised that clients had unmet medication needs, the nurses were unsure:

> who was responsible for monitoring side effects, ensuring clients' and carers' understanding of their prescribed medication and optimizing compliance with medication (Jordan et al., 1999).

In a study with practice nurses, Lowe and colleagues explored the effects of additional medication questions in the over-75 health check (Lowe et al., 2000). The practice nurse asked questions to correlate the medicines taken by the patient with the surgery records (including medicine, dose and frequency); ability to open the medicine packaging; ability to use non-oral devices; and any concerns regarding the medication. Using this set of screening questions the nurses found discrepancies between practice medication records and what the patient was actually taking in 65% of the 34 patients studied. In some cases the discrepancy was minor but in 10 patients it was judged clinically significant. Five patients were referred for 'complete medication review'. The additional questions took about 6 minutes to administer and were reported to be acceptable to both nurse and patients.

Our ongoing research on statins (Chatterton et al., 2004) confirms that, on the whole, community pharmacists do not engage in discussions with patients presenting repeat prescriptions. We are exploring with pharmacists their perceptions about who is responsible for monitoring treatment.

Repeat dispensing and the potential contribution of pharmacists

Research demonstrates that community pharmacists have less involvement in information- and advice-giving in relation to repeat prescriptions than first-time prescriptions. In a USA study of patients' attitudes towards pharmacist counselling on prescribed medicines, 70% said they had not been offered counselling by their pharmacist (Erickson *et al.*, 1998). In a USA study community pharmacists asked patients questions about their medicines in 32% of interactions, but only 16 of 82 questions asked were monitoring medicines use (Sleath, 1995).

A Canadian study of patients prescribed antidepressants found that fewer than half of the patients recalled any discussion with the pharmacist once the initial prescription had been dispensed. The responses of pharmacists in the study led the author to conclude that most community pharmacists did not review monitoring of response to treatment as part of their role. Interestingly, pharmacists rated the value of their communication more highly than did antidepressant users, suggesting a gap between pharmacists' and patients' perceptions of needs. Pharmacists felt that the major barrier to effective communication was lack of privacy (Gardner *et al.*, 2001). Our own research with community pharmacists on depression indicates that they tend not to engage in conversations with patients on repeat prescriptions for antidepressants (Landers *et al.*, 2002). Pharmacists expressed concerns that such discussions might conflict with what the doctor had told the patient (or indeed, what the doctor might want or not want the patient to be told). Although pharmacists' accounts suggested that the pharmacy premises and lack of privacy were issues, the potential for conflict with doctors was a more influential factor.

Some patients may be unsure or unenthusiastic about pharmacist monitoring of medication and a Dutch study found that, while 31% of patients said they would be happy to discuss their medicines with the pharmacist, 51% said they would not and the remainder were unsure. However, patients who had discussed their medicines with the pharmacist in the past said they would want to do so again (Beijer and Blaey, 1999). Where community pharmacist monitoring was provided for patients receiving antidepressants, the results showed that adherence and patient satisfaction increased (Bultman and Svarstad, 2002). A study of pharmacist consultations with patients in the setting of the general practice found that patients were willing to talk in detail with the pharmacist about their medicines (Chen and Britten, 2000). The influence of the setting on patients' views is unknown. The general practice offers greater privacy than many community pharmacies and the association of the pharmacist with the doctors may also be an important factor. Overall, the results of research to date suggest that many patients would welcome the pharmacist's intervention to provide further information.

In community pharmacy it has been suggested that repeat dispensing offers the greatest opportunity for pharmacists to become more involved in medication monitoring, and hence chronic disease management. Repeat dispensing is a system where the community pharmacist is authorised to dispense repeat medication without the need for the patient to visit the surgery. Theoretically, repeat dispensing offers the opportunity for the community pharmacist to take a more proactive input to treatment monitoring. Pilot studies in Scotland and England showed the service to be well received by patients, with a large majority saying they would use the service if it were offered in the future. However, the pilots were run differently, with the Scottish pharmacists using a short structured questioning protocol at each dispensing point (Bond *et al.*, 2000), while in the English pilot the pharmacists were left to decide the content of the interaction with the patient (Wilson *et al.*, 2002).

A minority of the patients in the English pilot (15%) agreed that their pharmacist 'regularly talked with them' prior to their joining the scheme. After the scheme 76% recalled being asked if all of their repeat medicines were required but only 10% remembered being asked if they had any side-effects and only 9% whether they had taken all of the medicines they had received on the previous occasion. Most (70%) had not noticed any change in the way they were dealt with by the pharmacist. Patients' positive response to the scheme was mainly accounted for by increased convenience and time saved.

The Scottish pilot included all adult patients receiving a repeat prescription, with the exclusion of the contraceptive pill, hormone replacement therapy and drugs for the treatment of drug dependency. The study found that a proportion were experiencing side-effects from treatment. Patient satisfaction levels were high (Jones *et al.*, 2000). A total of 12.4% of patients had compliance problems, side-effects, adverse drug reactions or drug interactions identified by the pharmacist. There were significantly more problems identified in total in the intervention group. Sixty-six per cent of the study patients did not require their full quota of prescribed drugs, representing 18% of the total prescribed costs (Bond *et al.*, 2000).

The results of these studies suggest that introducing a repeat dispensing service without an accompanying framework for pharmacist intervention may have little impact on patient care, although it would undoubtedly increase convenience for patients. However, they show again that a foundation already exists on which to build more indepth discussions to support concordance, which would be acceptable to both pharmacists and patients and fit into their daily routines.

Medication review

Medication review involves a more detailed, and systematic, exploration of the patient's use of medication. In England the National Service Framework for Older People requires that patients over the age of 75 have a medication review at least annually, and 6-monthly if they are taking four or more medicines (Department of Health, 2001). Implementation of this policy highlighted that there were different interpretations of what constituted a 'medication review' and that reviews were often not recorded on the computerised records, making it difficult to know whether one had been conducted.

A recent study of pharmacist-led, general practice-based medication review found that such review was effective and identified and solved more medication-related problems than the GP's usual care (Zermansky *et al.*, 2001).

As practice has evolved in operationalising medication review, the range of healthcare staff involved has expanded and models have emerged with a combination of doctors, pharmacists, nurses, pharmacy technicians and general practice administrative staff. Whilst some of these models are based solely on paper-based review of records, most involve patient contact, providing another opportunity to develop rapport and explore concordance-related issues.

A set of practical tools for medication review can be found in the Medicines Partnership Centre's Room for Review, which can be downloaded from www.medicines-partnership.org.

What support might be provided?

Information and advice

Verbal information

Pressures on doctors' time have led to suggestions that pharmacists and nurses could be responsible for providing information and answering patients' questions about medicines. The importance of finding out what the patient wants to know as well as providing information that the practitioner feels needs to be given has been highlighted earlier in this chapter. Nurses' and pharmacists' time is also limited and more creative ways need to be found to meet patients' needs. The key issue is how to make the most of the brief interactions that take place regularly between practitioner and patient as well as the longer consultations that can occur during medication review.

There is also the issue of how much information patients can recall following a discussion with a health professional. Experience suggests that the average number of information items recalled by patients is three to four. However, studies have usually focused on unsolicited information rather than that given in response to patients' own questions.

The use of 'agenda forms' is almost unexplored in discussions about medication. In McKinley's study of the use of written patient agendas in general practice consultations, patients were given a simple form asking them to list the points they wanted to raise and any questions they wanted to ask (McKinley and Middleton, 1999). Patients were given a written message asking them to write down questions for their pharmacist in a community pharmacy study of patients presenting a first-time prescription. The pharmacist then incorporated answers to these questions into his or her counselling (Barnett et al., 2000). Fifty-six of the 106 patients asked to write down their questions did so and 52 of these wanted to ask about side-effects. Patients who wrote down their questions subsequently took a more active part in the discussion with the pharmacist than those in the control group. However, patient recall and satisfaction were not significantly different in the intervention group, although the pharmacists were more satisfied with the information they gave.

The use of simple questioning can successfully elicit patients' further information needs. In a study of extended adherence support from community pharmacists for people with hypertension, a brief structured questioning protocol was the intervention used. Pharmacists asked how the patient was getting on with the medicines, about side-effects, compliance and whether the patient would like any more information about their medicines (Blenkinsopp et al., 2000). Information was provided verbally and in the form of a user-friendly illustrated booklet about hypertension. Patients with intolerable side-effects (about 10%) were referred to their doctor. Six months after the study blood pressure was more likely to be controlled in the intervention group.

Written information

Since 1999 a European directive has required that every dispensed medicine must be accompanied by a manufacturer's PIL. Currently this is the only information that a patient is guaranteed to receive. Soon after the mandatory policy was implemented, Bandesha *et al.* (1996) conducted a survey with 215 patients in England. Most (83%) said they had noticed the leaflet but 17% had not. Of those who had noticed, the leaflet 21% said they had read all of it and 40% had read at least some of it. The manufacturers' leaflets are likely to meet some of patients' information needs but cannot be tailored so that they relate to individual patients' conditions. Furthermore there are restrictions such that the PIL has to describe the possible side-effects of the treatment yet cannot describe the potential benefits.

Health literacy is an important determinant of whether written information can be assimilated and understood. Much of the research on health literacy comes from the USA and a major study involving interviews with 3260 people tested the participants on their understanding of prescription medicine labels, appointment slips and informed consent forms. The results showed that over one-third had inadequate or marginal health literacy and prescription instructions were often misread (Gazmararian *et al.*, 1999). These findings have implications for the use of PILs. Some pharmaceutical companies have introduced user testing as part of their leaflet development process but many PILs are thought to be inadequate.

Well-produced and user-friendly leaflets offer the potential to improve the consistency of information provided by different professionals. Use of the same information leaflets would be a helpful starting point and there are good examples of independently produced materials (see, for example, *Drug and Therapeutics Bulletin*/Consumer Association leaflets at www.which.net/health/dtb/treatment.html).

The internet

Inadequate and marginal health literacy is also relevant in relation to patients seeking information on the internet, where it interferes with individuals' capacity to conduct searches and access information as well as to read and interpret what is found.

Research on health-related use of the internet showed that users sought information to find out more about, and perhaps challenge, their prescribed treatment. Indeed, a number of participants reported that they had used information found on the net to renegotiate treatment for themselves or their children. Searches that were initially for information on medication often led to information on complementary therapies. The internet enabled people to explore potentially embarrassing or sensitive health topics that they might otherwise not have raised with a health professional (Hardey, 1999).

Health professionals are not always comfortable about patients' use of the internet to access health information. They have expressed concerns about the quality and accuracy of the information obtained from the net and there has been an emphasis on attempting to control information through 'approved' websites that meet health professionals' criteria. While there is value in attempts to increase the accuracy of information and make potential conflicts of interest more explicit (see, for example, Kim *et al.*, 1999), it is impossible to control the availability of information on the internet.

Patients recognise that health professionals are busy and that their time is limited. The internet offers a way for patients to access up-to-date health information about conditions and their treatment and fits with the Expert Patient concept. Practitioners can support patients by:

1. asking if they have accessed additional information and what they thought about what they found
2. becoming familiar with, and recommending, particular websites for specific conditions and treatments
3. not being dismissive or judgemental about information that patients bring to the consultation

Patients as teachers

Making greater use of patients as a resource for other patients is a key component for the future (Wykura and Kelly, 2002). In England the Expert Patient movement is growing with support from the NHS, and a national programme of training courses in self-management is underway. The trainers are patients themselves and the aim of the courses is to enable patients to set goals and to cope better with their chronic condition.

Prompts and reminders

Patients devise their own systems to help them to remember to take their medicines and to be sure that they have taken them. Pharmacists and nurses can support this by using, for example, charts and calendars. Simple paper-based tools such as medicines reminder charts have been shown to increase compliance. Such charts can have a set of columns for dose times and a row for each medicine. In addition to the medicine's name the chart can indicate what it does and whether the dose is to be taken regularly or as needed. Changes in technology have enabled direct communication prompts using, for example, mobile phone text messaging and e-mail. Different approaches will suit different patients and can be tailored to the patient's preference.

Multicompartment compliance aids

Various box-type devices have been designed to serve as a medication container, as a reminder mechanism, and to provide a check that doses have been taken. These multicompartment compliance aids (MCAs) usually hold a week's supply of the patient's medicines in small compartments. Their use may be initiated by patients, carers, hospitals, social services staff and primary care practitioners. There is little evidence of their effectiveness but nevertheless they are widely used.

One study aimed to determine the scale of dispensing into compliance aids by community pharmacists, how the service was provided and the extent to which it met patients' needs (Nunney and Raynor, 2001). Over three-quarters of community pharmacists reported dispensing into MCAs for some of their patients (mean 11, range 1–70). The most commonly used MCAs were Nomad (52%) and Dosett (27%). In an accompanying qualitative study, eight of 10 pharmacists interviewed said they supplied their preferred device without reference to the patient. Fifty-six patients were interviewed in the study and more than two-thirds did not know the names of their medicines, while one in five reported difficulty in using the MCA. The authors conclude that large numbers of patients living at home have their medicines dispensed in an MCA and in that in most cases this was initiated without an assessment of their needs.

A considerable amount of resource (pharmacist and staff time) is being used to provide a service with uncertain outcomes and benefits. Dispensing prescription medicines into an MCA is a time-consuming process for the community pharmacist and has to be done weekly (compared to the more usual monthly or 2-monthly supply) and until recently the pharmacist has generally received no payment for this work. In 2002 an NHS scheme was introduced in Scotland to limit the use of such aids to those with identified need, not demand. The scheme involves patient referral from primary care practitioners to an accredited pharmacist, followed by a standard assessment carried out by the pharmacist. This includes consideration of options other than an MCA to the meet the patient's need. Appropriate professional fees are paid to the pharmacist for both the assessment and ongoing supply.

The future

While research evidence indicates the promise of positive effects on patient care resulting from pharmacist and nurse support for medication use, the practice models are not yet widely used. Supplementary prescribing (www.doh.gov.uk/supplementaryprescribing) will provide an opportunity for nurses, pharmacists and other healthcare professionals more actively to monitor and review treatment.

For routine nursing and pharmacy practice, learning simple models for using questions to elicit patients' views and enable discussion about treatment could be introduced in basic or post basic training. For pharmacists, such learning would supplement their existing knowledge and skills in pharmacology and therapeutics. For nursing, the needs are likely to be different. A review of the adequacy of the educational preparation of nurses for a medication role highlighted the importance of clarifying outcomes and competencies required as well as ensuring sufficient taught pharmacology and practice-based learning (Latter *et al.*, 2000).

The introduction of repeat dispensing in the UK brings an opportunity to enhance treatment monitoring as well as increase convenience and save time for patients. It would be a pity if this opportunity were not taken.

Harnessing the skills and expertise of patients as teachers and supporters of other patients is perhaps the most powerful tool for change in the future. Enabling patients to assume as much responsibility as they wish for their own treatment will require partnership working by health professionals and the sharing of power. Health professionals will need to rise to this challenge and see it as an opportunity rather than a threat.

This chapter has set out some ways in which health professionals can, as part of their routine practice, work with patients towards greater concordance in medicine-taking. It has shown that the prescribing decision is not the only place where action can be taken to enhance concordance. In the postprescription phase pharmacists and nurses have a particularly important contribution to make in listening and responding to patients' beliefs about medicines and their experiences of medicine-taking.

References

Bandesha G, Raynor D K, Teale C (1996). Preliminary investigation of patient information leaflets as package inserts. *Int J Pharm Pract* 4: 246–248.

Barnett C W, Nykamp D, Ellington A M (2000). Patient-guided counselling in the community pharmacy setting. *J Am Pharm Assoc* 40 (6): 765–772.

Barry C A, Bradley C P, Britten N *et al.* (2000). Patients' unvoiced agendas in general practice consultations: qualitative study. *BMJ* 320: 1236–1250; erratum *BMJ* 321: 44.

Beijer H J M, De Blaey C J (1999). An instrument to trace medication problems. The results of the Dutch hypertension week. *Pharmaceutisch Weekblad* 134 (34): 1182–1185.

Benson J, Britten N (2002). Patients' decisions about whether or not to take antihypertensive drugs: qualitative study. *BMJ* 325: 873–876.

Berg J S, Dischler J, Wagner D J *et al.* (1993). Medication compliance: a healthcare problem. *Ann Pharmacother* 27: S1–S24.

Berry D C, Michas I C, Gillie A, Forster M (1997). What do patients want to know about their medicines and what do doctors want to tell them? A comparative study. *Psychol Health* 12: 467–480.

Blenkinsopp A, Phelan M, Bourne J, Dakhil N (2000). Extended adherence support by community pharmacists for patients with hypertension: a randomized controlled trial. *Int J Pharm Pract* 8: 165–175.

Blom L, Jonkers R, Kok G, Bakker A (1998). Patient education in 20 Dutch community pharmacies. *Int J Pharm Pract* 6 (2): 72–76.

Bond C, Matheson C, Williams S *et al.* (2000). Repeat prescribing: a role for community pharmacists in controlling and monitoring repeat prescriptions. *Br J Gen Pract* 50 (453): 271–275.

Bultman D C, Svarstad B L (2002). Effects of pharmacist monitoring on patient satisfaction with antidepressant medication therapy. *J Am Pharm Assoc* 42: 36–43.

Chatterton M, Blenkinsopp A, Pollock K (2004). Statins and the interface between patient and community pharmacist. Health Services Research and Pharmacy Practice Conference, London, 2004. Available online at: http://hsrpp.org.uk/abstracts/2004_03.shtml (accessed 16 April 2004).

Chen J, Britten N (2000). 'Strong medicine': an analysis of pharmacist consultations in primary care. *Fam Pract* 17: 480–483.

Chewning B, Schommer J (1996). Increasing clients' knowledge of community pharmacists' roles. *Pharm Res* 13: 1299–1304.

Cox K, Stevenson F, Britten N, Dundar Y (2004). A systematic review of communication between health professionals and patients about medicine-taking and prescribing. Available online at www.medicines-partnership.org/research-evidence/major-reviews/systematic-review (accessed 16 April 2004).

Department of Health (2001). *Implementing Medicines-Related Aspects of the Older People NSF.* London: Department of Health.

Erickson S R, Kirking D M, Sandusky M (1998). Michigan Medicaid recipients' perceptions of medication counseling as required by OBRA 90. *J Am Pharm Assoc* 38: 333–338.

Gardner D M, Murphy A L, Woodman A K, Connelly S (2001). Community pharmacy services for antidepressant users. *Int J Pharm Pract* 9: 217–224.

Gazmararian J A, Baker D W, Williams M V *et al.* (1999). Health literacy among Medicare enrollees in a managed care organization. *JAMA* 281: 545–551.

Hardey M (1999). Doctor in the house: the internet as a source of lay health knowledge and the challenge to expertise. *Sociol Health Ill* 21: 820–835.

Houghton J,Woods F, Davis S *et al.* (1999). Community pharmacist reporting of suspected adverse drug reactions: (2) Attitudes of community pharmacists and general practitioners in Wales. *Pharm J* 263: 788–791.

Hughes M L, Whittlesea C M C, Luscombe D K (2002). Symptom or ADR? An investigation into how symptoms are recognized as side effects of medication. *Pharm J* 269: 719–722.

Jones J, Matheson C, Bond C M (2000). Patients' satisfaction with a novel method to control repeat prescribing. *IJPP* 8 (4): 291–297.

Jordan S, Hardy B, Coleman M (1999). Medication management: an exploratory study into the role of community mental health nurses. *J Adv Nurs* 29 (5): 1068–1081.

Kim P, Eng T R, Deering M J, Maxfield A (1999). Published criteria for evaluating health related web sites: review. *BMJ* 318: 647–649.

Landers M, Blenkinsopp A, Pollock K, Grime J (2002). Community pharmacists and depression: the pharmacist as intermediary between patient and GP. *Int J Pharm Pract* 10: 253–265.

Latter S, Rycroft-Malone J, Yerrell P, Shaw D (2000). Evaluating educational preparation for a health education role in practice: the case of medication education. *J Adv Nurs* 32 (5): 1282–1290.

Lip G Y, Beevers D G (1996). A survey of the current practice of treating hypertension in primary care: the Rational Evaluation and Choice in Hypertension (REACH) study. *J Drug Dev Clin Pract* 8: 161–169.

Lip G Y, Beevers D G (1997). Doctors, nurses, pharmacists and patients – the Rational Evaluation and Choice in Hypertension (REACH) survey of hypertension care delivery. *Blood Pressure Suppl* (1): 6–10.

Livingstone C R (1996). Verbal interactions between elderly people and community pharmacists about prescription medication. *Int J Pharm Pract* 4: 12–18.

Livingstone C R, Pugh A L G, Winn S, Williams V K (1996). Developing community pharmacy services wanted by local people: information and advice about prescription medicines. *Int J Pharm Pract* 4: 94–102.

Lowe C J, Raynor D K, Teale C, Lubgan G (2000). Can practice nurses identify medication problems using the over-75 health check? *J Clin Nurs* 9: 816–817.

McKinley R F, Middleton J F (1999). What do patients want from doctors? Content analysis of written patient agendas for the consultation. *Br J Gen Pract* 49: 796–800.

Montbriand M J (2000). Senior and health professionals' perceptions and communication about prescriptions and alternative therapies. *Can J Ageing* 19: 35–56.

Nunney J M, Raynor D K (2001). How are multi-compartment compliance aids used in primary care? *Pharm J* 267: 784–789.

Royal Pharmaceutical Society of Great Britain (1997). *From Compliance to Concordance: Achieving Shared Goals in Medicine Taking.* London: RPSGB.

Savage I (1997). Time for prescription and over the counter advice in independent community practice. *Int J Pharm Pract* 258: 873–877.

Savage I (1999). The changing face of pharmacy practice – evidence from 20 years of work sampling studies. *Int J Pharm Pract* 7: 209–219.

Schafheutle E, Hassell K, Seston E M, Noyce P R (2002). Non-dispensing of NHS prescriptions. *Int J Pharm Pract* 10: 11–16.

Sleath B (1995). Pharmacist question-asking in New Mexico community pharmacies. *Am J Pharm Ed* 59: 374–379.

Sleath B, Chewning B, Svarstad B, Roter D (2000). Patient expression of complaints and adherence problems with medications during chronic disease medical visits. *J Soc Admin Pharm* 17: 71–80.

Wilson K A, Jesson J K, Varnish J *et al.* (2002). The Birmingham community pharmacy repeat dispensing project. *Pharm J* 269: 20–24.

Wykura G, Kelly D (2002). Developing the role of patients as teachers. *BMJ* 325: 818–821.

Zermansky A G, Petty D R, Raynor D K *et al.* (2001). Randomised controlled trial of clinical medication review by a pharmacist of elderly patients receiving repeat prescriptions in general practice. *BMJ* 323 (7325): 1340–1343.

6

Educational perspectives on concordance

Marjorie Weiss

Introduction

There is a nebulous quality about concordance. While it has been described and elaborated, discussed and debated, misconstrued and derided, it lacks a precision in terms of what it practically means health-care professionals should be *doing* in their interactions with patients. Further, it is a concept that needs to be both flexible and adaptable to a broad range of encounters with patients, yet able to evolve over time as our thinking progresses. Developing an educational strategy that is able to embrace this dual nature of concordance, with its amorphous and diverse qualities, is indeed a substantial undertaking.

None the less, a lack of definitional certainty in terms of practical application is not only confined to concordance. Other related concepts, such as shared decision-making, patient partnership and patient-centredness, enjoy a similar contested character as to how they can be actually implemented in practice. These concepts also provide a valuable insight into how concordance can be taught. For this reason, information in this chapter has been drawn from a range of sources in the physician, nursing and pharmacy literature. This chapter reports some of the literature exploring, for example using the medical paradigm, doctor–patient communication, doctor–patient interactions or the doctor–patient relationship. It draws upon work using conceptual frameworks such as shared decision-making, patient-centredness, effective communication and humanistic interactions. It explores how these issues have been taught in a range of clinical areas, most notably in the area of palliative care. The aim here is not to review all these areas systematically but briefly to discuss some of the key issues.

In the nursing literature Wilkinson (1991) has defined effective communication as open two-way communication in which patients are informed about the nature of their disease and treatment and are encouraged to express their anxieties and emotions. Concordance has a degree of commonality with this, yet seems to take this idea a stage further, to include both a negotiated outcome between professional and patient, and the option for follow-up, should that be desired. Conceptually, concordance is closely allied to the shared model of treatment decision-making that promotes active patient involvement in the decision-making process (Charles *et al.*, 1999). In Charles' model (taking the physician perspective), the four necessary characteristics for a shared approach are:

1.   Both the physician and patient are involved in the treatment decision-making process.
2.   Both the physician and patient share information with each other.
3.   Both the physician and patient take steps to participate in the decision-making process by expressing treatment preferences.
4.   A treatment decision is made and both the physician and patient agree on the treatment to implement.

This conceptual 'map' for the shared model of treatment decision-making provides a basis for teaching and learning in concordance. The perspective taken in this chapter is that concordance follows the shared model of decision-making as applied to medicine-taking. The issues identified have relevance for the teaching and learning of all healthcare professionals – doctors, pharmacists and nurses.

What do we want to teach?

The practice of concordance requires the healthcare professional to develop appropriate skills, knowledge and attitudes. The following sections consider these issues, taking a practice-based approach to the implementation of concordance. This section considers educational issues unique to concordance where basic clinical knowledge is assumed.

Skills

At the heart of the practice of concordance lies the implementation of communication skills. For this reason, a predominantly skills-based approach to the teaching and learning of concordance is entirely appropriate. The types of skills needed have been discussed by previous authors (Kurtz *et al.*, 1998; Hargie *et al.*, 2000; Smith *et al.*, 2000; Makoul, 2001) and various frameworks, algorithms and acronyms devised to act as *aide-mémoires*. The key components are, however, common to most, if not all, of these and may be summarised as follows:

- Greeting – appropriate initial greeting and introductions ensures patient comfort and privacy, identifies the issues the patient wants to address.
- Exploring – elicits the patient's view of his or her health and illness, explores the patient's psychosocial and emotional issues such as the impact of the health problem on his or her life, discusses patient's expectations.
- Questioning – uses open questions where possible, avoids leading questions.
- Listening – giving patients the learner's undivided attention, does not interrupt the patient, picks up verbal and non-verbal cues.
- Empathising and supporting – encourages patient to ask questions, probes and facilitates patient responses, acknowledges patient views and concerns, demonstrates appropriate non-verbal behaviour (e.g. open body posture, head-nodding and forward-leaning).
- Clarifying and summarising patient responses – checks own understanding of issues.
- Sharing information – shares thinking with patient to encourage patient involvement, avoids the use of jargon, provides rationale for any examination needed, provides information on treatment choices and possible side-effects in a comprehensible manner, checks patient's level of understanding.
- Agreeing the issues with the patient – elicits patient's reactions and feelings to the information provided, encourages patient responses, negotiates a mutually acceptable plan, discusses the patient's ability to follow the plan (e.g. time constraints, how it fits into his or her life).
- Concluding and planning – summarises outcome of interaction, explores whether there is anything else the patient wants to discuss, agrees next steps with patient, discusses what to do if something goes wrong.

Knowledge

Underpinning the development of a skills base in concordance is the knowledge base that provides the rationale for the importance of the subject area. In this respect the three key issues for knowledge-based learning in concordance are:

1. the meaning of concordance and its relevance for practice
2. the historical development of concordance and its evolution from compliance
3. the evidence in favour of a concordant approach and the need for it as part of routine practice

Information exploring issues such as the development of concordance and the cost and health consequences of non-compliance can be obtained from other chapters of this book. However, other useful sources include an interview with Marshall Marinker on the meaning of concordance (Marinker, 2000), Stewart's (1995) review of effective communication and health outcomes, Mead and Bower's (2000) review of patient-centredness, a review of the literature in doctor–patient communication (Ong *et al.*, 1995) and an evaluation of communication-training programmes in nursing care (Kruijver *et al.*, 2000). To promote discussion on the question of whether a concordant approach will take more time, there is an article by Marvel *et al.* (1999) on the extent to which physicians elicited patient concerns in the consultation. This study found that patients who were allowed to complete their statement of concerns used only 6 seconds more on average that those who were redirected (interrupted) before completion occurred (Marvel *et al.*, 1999). In addition, there is the study by Britten *et al.* (2000) on some of the misunderstandings, and consequent adverse health outcomes, that occur in general practice when doctors and patients miscommunicate. Of particular interest is a recent Cochrane review of interventions for providers to promote a patient-centred approach in the clinical consultation. This review concluded that there is limited and mixed evidence on the effects of such interventions on patient healthcare behaviours or health status. However, it is likely that some interventions promoting patient-centred care lead to significant improvements in consultation processes and may positively impact upon patient satisfaction with care (Lewin *et al.*, 2002).

Attitudes

Skills-based training and the provision of knowledge may only partly address an individual healthcare professional's learning needs to implement concordance. Blocks to poor communication may not relate purely to skills but may relate to the healthcare professional's beliefs about the roles of patients and healthcare professionals in the therapeutic process (Kurtz *et al.*, 1998: 35). Concepts such as caring, respect for the patient, comfort and trust fall within this affective domain and represent important themes which must be addressed as part of any training in concordance. This can be problematic for educators, as it may be easier to focus on the more tangible, task-focused skills training than on the development of attitudes appropriate to the concordant approach.

To convey positive affective attributes, healthcare professionals need greater awareness of the influence of their personal style on the nature of their interactions with patients. Authors have advocated the need for professionals to reflect upon their own personal characteristics and the effects these can have on communication with patients (Branch *et al.*, 2001; DiBartola, 2001). Branch *et al.* (2001) argue that health-care professionals need to be aware of the emotions evoked in the context of a patient interaction. This awareness includes recognition of one's values, beliefs, history, needs and culture. This is comparable to Mead and Bower's (2000) dimension of 'doctor as person' in their description of the patient-centred model. In this description, patient-centred medicine is 'two-person medicine' where doctor subjectivity is inherent in the doctor–patient relationship. Greater awareness of this influence can act as a stimulus to change, enabling an alteration of behaviour and improvements to the care of the patient. As noted by DiBartola, all professionals have a preferred communication style and, once recognised, it is possible for an individual to adapt his or her style better to suit the needs of the patient (DiBartola, 2001).

Negative affective responses can result from a concern that greater inquiry into personal issues may result in increased patient distress or may threaten the healthcare professional's own emotional survival (Maguire and Pitceathly, 2002). For this reason emotional cues provided in the consultation by the patient may result in blocking behaviour which discourages further disclosure. These blocking behaviours include: offering advice and reassurance before the main problems have been identified; explaining away distress as normal; attending to physical aspects only; switching the topic or 'jollying' patients along (Maguire and Pitceathly, 2002).

The influence of personal values, beliefs and attitudes on the nature of the professional–patient interaction has led some authors to advocate for greater training in these issues. Novack *et al.* (1997) has outlined a training programme for medical students to achieve greater personal awareness and effective patient care. This programme contains four core topics. Firstly, the programme includes an exploration of physicians' beliefs and attitudes such as core beliefs, personal philosophy and family influences. Secondly, physicians' feelings and emotional responses in patient care, particularly focusing on love and anger, are discussed. The third area of challenging clinical situations includes dealing with difficult patients and dying patients and handling medical mistakes. Finally, the programme includes physician self-care such as balancing personal and professional lives and managing stress (Novack *et al.*, 1997). A programme focusing on similar issues would be appropriate for the development of concordance. From this evidence, it is possible to identify three key attitudinal attributes integral to the practice of concordance:

1. the demonstration of empathy and caring in the interaction
2. respect for the patient's view
3. self-awareness of one's personal values, beliefs and history and how these shape the professional–patient relationship

Objectives

Many authors have described the aims and objectives for involving patients in decisions about their health. Much research has developed from the medical paradigm that has relevance for all healthcare professionals. For example, Elwyn *et al.* (2000) have described the various competences necessary for involving patients in healthcare choices. Similarly, Towle and Godolphin (1999) have discussed competencies for the practice of informed shared decision-making by physicians and patients while Branch *et al.* (2001) have reviewed various educational strategies for teaching the humanistic dimensions of care during medical education. Edwards and Elwyn (2001) draw a distinction between competencies and competences. *Competencies* are innate personal attributes enabling learning while *competences* are situational and task-linked skills which can be learnt. Both are needed in the practice of concordance.

Coté and Leclere (2000) have organised their competencies for describing doctor–patient relationships by skill level. In this respect, at level 1 are those skills necessary for conducting the interview effectively and politely. Level 2 skills are those necessary for understanding and involving the patient and level 3 skills are those necessary for managing emotionally complex situations. This approach of different skill levels appropriate to the needs and experience of the learner can be applied to concordance. The four 'core' aims necessary for the teaching and learning of concordance can be described as follows:

1. Builds a relationship with the patient through the use of good verbal and non-verbal communication skills.
2. Elicits the patient's concerns, expectations and beliefs about his or her condition and its treatment.
3. Provides clinical information in a manner appropriate to the patient.
4. Involves the patient in an agreed management plan.

However, these are broad aims for learning which may be met through the achievement of different levels of objectives depending upon the skills and experience of the learner. The aims and different levels of objectives for teaching are shown in Table 6.1.

For example, level 1 objectives may be appropriate for an entry-level undergraduate pharmacy, nursing or medical student. Level 2 might be appropriate for later undergraduate or postgraduate students. Level 3 might be appropriate for postgraduate students or those already in practice as part of continuing professional development. It should be noted that all the levels of teaching are cumulative, such that should a learner have a target to meet the level 3 objective for building a relationship, then it is assumed that s/he is already proficient in levels 1 and 2 in that issue. Further, these levels are not rigid, such that a learner might be a level 2 in one issue while a level 1 in another. In this sense, the objectives for teaching a particular issue in concordance need to be tailored to the individual needs and experience of the learner. Particularly for earlier levels of teaching, it may be appropriate to provide the relevant clinical information, reminding students that the purpose of the learning exercise is to focus on the core concordance skills, not on the clinical information.

A complementary approach is to view the healthcare professional–patient consultation as an event with an inherent chronology, concentrating on the skills needed early in the consultation in earlier years of the healthcare professional's training. This approach would see the process of gathering information at the beginning of a consultation to be the main focus of early concordance skills training when the learner lacks clinical knowledge. This approach has been used in medical school training with first- and second-year undergraduates. Students are taught basic information-gathering skills, presented in the guise of needing to acquire patient information as part of a medical history that is to be summarised and fed back to the senior consultant. For pharmacists, such an approach would be analogous to taking a patient's medication history as part of the process of pharmaceutical care (James *et al.*, 2001). Authors have advocated placing an emphasis on initiating the session, including gathering information (focusing on initial exploration of the patient's problem and exploration of the patient's perspective of the illness), building a relationship with the patient, summarising the session and communicating with a diversity of patients (Laidlaw *et al.*, 2002). Skills used in the later stages of the consultation, such as providing information in a manner appropriate for the patient and involving the patient in an agreed management plan, can be taught in

Table 6.1 Core concordance aims with objective levels

Aims	Potential objective levels (dependent upon learner's previous training and experience)		
	Level 1	Level 2	Level 3
1. Builds a relationship with the patient through the use of good verbal and non-verbal communication skills	Ensures appropriateness of the environment (e.g. privacy). Listens without interruption. Uses open questions. Displays appropriate body language	Structures the consultation in a logical sequence. Displays empathy and rapport through the use of probes and facilitative responses. Ensures appropriate follow-up	Displays self-awareness of the patient's personal values and the impact these can have upon the relationship
2. Elicits the patient's concerns, expectations and beliefs about his or her condition and its treatment	Asks patient if there is anything else he or she would like to discuss	Acknowledges patient's concerns. Picks up on patient cues that occur in the consultation	Fully explores patient's concerns, explicitly recognising the patient's expertise in how his or her body responds to illness
3. Provides clinical information in a manner appropriate to the patient	Avoids the use of jargon and presents information in a clear and concise manner	Ascertains if the patient would like more information and, if so, in what format (e.g. text, drawings, bar charts, numbers)	Relates clinical explanations to patient's previously elicited concerns or beliefs
4. Involves the patient in an agreed management plan	Suggests the best way forward and obtains agreement from the patient	Ascertains if the patient would like to be involved in decision-making. Professional shares his or her thoughts on what s/he thinks are the important issues for making a decision about management	Reviews and evaluates complex clinical and psychosocial information with the patient. Helps patient reflect on the impact of alternative decisions on his or her life and which options are consistent with the patient's personal values

the later years of training when more clinical knowledge has been acquired.

How will it be taught?

While a variety of educational methods may be used to facilitate the learning of concordance skills, knowledge and attitudes, a learner-centred approach should be an important component of this teaching and learning. A learner-centred approach facilitates learners' identification of their own needs and interests and leads to attitudes of self-efficacy, as well as a greater sense of autonomy and self-direction (Knowles, 1980). Active learning puts a high priority on the skills learners need to acquire or to refine in order to make use of what they know (Denicolo et al., 1992). It involves giving learners greater responsibility for their own learning – for them to be challenged to think things through for themselves, to identify and tackle problems and to share and discuss ideas with others (Revans, 1982: 626–627). Kaufman (2003), in his excellent review exploring the link between educational theory and teaching practice, describes seven principles to guide teaching practice which have emerged from these theories. These seven principles may be summarised as follows (Kaufman, 2003):

1. The learner should be an active contributor to the educational process.
2. Learning should closely relate understanding to solving real-life problems.
3. Learners' current knowledge and experience are critical. These should be taken into account in new learning situations.
4. Learners should be given the opportunity and support to use self-direction in their learning.
5. Learners should be given opportunities and support for practice, to include self-assessment and constructive feedback from teachers and peers.
6. Learners should be given the opportunity to reflect on their practice by analysing and assessing their own performance.
7. Use of role models by educators can have a major impact on learners as people often teach the way they were themselves taught.

In addition, as explained by Smith et al. (2000), learner-centred learning is the teaching counterpart of the patient-centred approach being taught. Mirroring a key theme of concordance to elicit and address the patient's view, the learner-centred approach recognises the importance of identifying and meeting learners' teaching and learning needs. As such, the emphasis on this section is not to identify one ideal approach but rather to give readers a 'toolkit' of methods from which to choose.

While didactic methods have been the traditional teaching approach, it has come under considerable criticism as unlikely to influence healthcare professionals' behaviour (Davis *et al.*, 1995). In this context, didactic methods are defined as an educational intervention consisting of a predominantly lecture or presentation format by a person in authority to a group of essentially passive listeners. A recent Cochrane review found that in six out of the 10 educational interventions using interactive workshops there were moderate or moderately large changes in professional practice (Thomson O'Brien *et al.*, 2004). In 12 out of 19 interventions that combined workshops and didactic presentations, moderate to moderately large changes in professional practice were identified. As noted by Branch *et al.* (2001), active learning approaches, which engage learners in doing, discussing and reflecting, more effectively promote humanistic skills, attitudes and values than do passive approaches, where learners simply observe another person's interactions. However, this is not to imply that didactic approaches have no role in the teaching and learning of concordance. Didactic sessions, in combination with more interactive approaches, can have a role in acquiring knowledge-based learning. In a unique study of the effectiveness of two guideline dissemination strategies in community pharmacy, Watson *et al.* (2002) found that neither an educational workshop nor an educational outreach visit was effective in changing community pharmacy staff behaviour. Watson *et al.*'s (2002) study reiterates the importance of focusing on professional behaviour change, not just an increase in a professional's knowledge, as the crucial outcome when assessing the impact of educational interventions. Further, it suggests that there could be other barriers inherent to community pharmacy which may inhibit behaviour change – and that these barriers may similarly be relevant for the implementation of concordance.

Kurtz *et al.* (1998: 56) suggest that learners can assimilate cognitive information as a part skills-based work when they can:

1. discover for themselves a need for information
2. actively grapple with the information rather than listen passively to its presentation
3. understand the rationale and principles behind the information rather than simply learn it by rote
4. understand the logical interconnections and the links between different pieces of information
5. group together various concepts into memorable categories
6. relate the information to its practical application

Lectures are particularly useful at the beginning of a workshop, offering a gentle introduction before beginning more active or experiential-based learning. A lecture can be used to describe the programme and overall goals for the workshop. This could be prefaced with pre-workshop assignments to read papers on the meaning of concordance or critically review the evidence in favour of a concordant approach. These assignments can be used as the basis for facilitating interaction in small group discussion after the didactic introduction. Kinmonth *et al.* (1996), in their training programme for GPs and nurses in patient-centred consulting, used brainstorming to compare professional-centred versus patient-centred approaches. Tiberius (1999) has reviewed a range of interactive methods suitable for small-group teaching as well as how to manage some common problems. Various small-group approaches are shown in Box 6.1.

One popular method used to promote discussion and critical reflection of a learner's skill base is to use narrative. As explained by Greenhalgh and Hurwitz (1999), narrative, or storytelling, has three components. A narrative has a finite and longitudinal time sequence; it presupposes both a narrator and a listener whose different viewpoints affect how the story is told; and it concerns how individuals feel and how people feel about them (Greenhalgh and Hurwitz, 1999). In relation to education, narrative can reveal worlds that are otherwise closed to us – such as those of the profoundly physically and mentally sick or patients of a different age, gender or ethnicity to ourselves (Greenhalgh, 2001). Importantly, stories can be used to help us reflect critically upon our professional practice. When practitioners help each other to think about cases, it can improve clinical care, developing practitioners' overall skills in questioning and reflection, and boosts their morale (Launer, 2002: 103). As a teaching tool in concordance, narrative can help learners reflect upon their practice through the use of structured prompts for relating a participant's story (Centre for Pharmacy Postgraduate Education, 2002). This series of prompts contains the following elements:

- a description of who and what the story is about
- why the story was chosen
- how the people felt or reacted
- whether anything should have been done differently
- learning points of the story for other people

Learners, having received the storytelling guide prior to an educational session, bring their story to the session. These stories are then used as

---

Box 6.1 Small-group methods to encourage student participation

Free group discussion
Sets a preplanned agenda, sets topics and assigned material to be covered. The group leader encourages everyone to participate and ensures the group does not drift too far from the agenda

Buzz groups
The small group is divided into groups of two or three. The groups are given a task and a time limit and a student records and feeds back their progress to the larger group. These types of groups are usually set up and run spontaneously within a larger group session

Learning cells
Two or three students read the material, answer set questions on their own and then discuss their answers with the group. This maximises active participation. This can be used in relation to a specific patient case study (patient-oriented problem-solving) or may be used to cover more general issues. Learning cells are usually run in conjunction with an assignment where students are given the task and feed back the results a day or several days later

Brain-storming
Members 'storm' a problem and come up with ideas. No criticism is allowed of contributions – all ideas are accepted and written down

Debate
This requires a controversial issue on which group members can take opposing sides. It has a formal structure (argument, opposing argument, rebuttal) where everyone is given a chance to speak

Reproduced with permission from Tiberius (1999).

---

part of small-group work where learners can listen to each other's stories, using the stories as a vehicle for identifying areas of learning need and reflecting on the important issues for practice.

Another possible approach is to use 'trigger' tapes. These can be in the form of simulated encounters (actor-patient and actor-professional), partially simulated encounters (actor-patient visiting professional/ learner) or actual encounters the participant has recorded prior to attending the workshop. These 'trigger' tapes form the basis of discussion and feedback in subsequent sessions. For example, in an evaluation of a communication skills-training programme for nurses in elderly care by Caris-Verhallen *et al.* (2000), the authors used video interaction analysis before and after skills training to assess the performance of nurses. Pairs of trainees, guided by their trainer, watched and discussed videotapes of their own performance during the training sessions. Roter *et al.* (1995) used audiotapes of actual patients in medical visits with physician participants as part of their training programme. Participants were asked to tape themselves practising their new skills with an actual patient and to identify one or two 5-minute segments from their tapes as the basis for discussion in the follow-up training session.

Role-play

A technique meriting particular note is the use of role-play. A role-play needs to be distinguished from acting. Acting consists of bringing to life a dramatist's ideas (or one's own ideas) in order to influence and entertain an audience. In contrast, role-play is the process of experiencing a problem under an unfamiliar set of constraints in order to stimulate one's own ideas and increase one's own understanding of a situation (Van Ments, 1989). Although sometimes disparaged by learners, when done correctly it provides an opportunity for learners to practise their skills, thereby enhancing learning. As some learners can find role-plays daunting it is important to establish the safety of the role-play environment. Before beginning, facilitators should acknowledge the unreality of the role-play situation and that its main purpose is to serve as a catalyst for learning for all concerned, not just the role-players. Experimentation by role-players is not only appreciated, but cherished. It is an opportunity to make mistakes in safety, to be immune from causing harm and to replay interviews again and again, something that never happens in real life (Kurtz *et al.*,1998). Learners may also need to be reminded that the purpose of the role-play is to practise skills; they should avoid concentrating too much on the clinical details.

Two basic techniques in role-play are the fishbowl and multiple techniques (Van Ments, 1989). Usually, the teacher/facilitator prepares the background information on the roles of professional and patient. In the fishbowl technique the principal players act out the role-play with the remainder of the group sitting around them in a circle. This observer group provides descriptive feedback at the end of the scenario. In the multiple technique, learners can act out the role-plays in parallel in small groups of three to four with additional members acting as observers and providing feedback. The role of the patient may be a 'model' patient or actor, or another student taking the role of patient. Boxes 6.2–6.4 give details of possible role-plays that could be used for pharmacists, doctors and nurses.

These scenarios are only examples of the types of situations that could be devised to develop learning in concordance. Additional contextual and clinical information may be added to provide a fuller description for the role-players. Underlying the design of these role-plays are the following features:

Box 6.2 Pharmacist–customer role-play example

Pharmacist's perspective

Mr Don Mullen comes into your pharmacy with a repeat prescription for omeprazole 20 mg daily for 1 month. Looking at your computerised patient medication record (PMR), you notice that Mr Mullen collected his initial prescription (30 days' supply) just over 3 months ago. Now he is returning for his second supply.

You would like to talk to Mr Mullen about his medicine-taking. Clinically, you recognise that omeprazole probably does not need to be taken longer than one daily for 2 months unless the patient has recurring symptoms. If he is experiencing further symptoms, you know it is best to take the omeprazole regularly to avoid rebound hyperacidity. What would you now like to say to Mr Mullen?

Patient's perspective

You are Don Mullen, a 34-year-old manager of a local branch of a grocery store chain. Approximately 5 months ago, you suffered from indigestion pains that were severe enough to result in several days off sick from work. This was of concern to you as you are quite a dedicated employee with a young family to support. At that time you saw Dr Jones, your local GP, and he prescribed some tablets. You have been pleased with how effective these tablets have been in getting rid of your indigestion. After starting the tablets, your symptoms have returned at odd intervals and the tablets have always helped. Upon occasion, the pain during these intervals has been severe enough for you to double the dose but then, in between these bouts, you stop taking the tablets.

Your main concern is that you want to make sure you have enough of the tablets should the pain get very severe again. Yet you also do not want to get addicted to the tablets and figure taking the tablets off and on is better than taking them all the time.

You are quite keen to know more about these tablets – for example, how they work, if they are addictive and if there are any side-effects. You consider yourself quite an independent person – quite used to managing by yourself any medical problem you might have.

Box 6.3 General practitioner–patient role-play example

General practitioner's perspective
Mrs Rose Smith is a 50-year-old patient of yours who was diagnosed with chronic myeloid leukaemia 1 year ago. She is under the care of the local hospital cancer specialist and appears to be responding well to the treatment. She comes today with the symptoms of a sore throat – her throat is inflamed and she has a bit of a cough. The symptoms have been present for a few days, although she does not have a fever. Her lymph nodes are not swollen and she has no tonsillar exudates. Given her clinical presentation, the practice's local antibiotic policy would be not to prescribe an antibiotic. Mrs Smith tells you she would like some antibiotics and appears quite worried. You have known her for a number of years and are quite sympathetic to her situation.

Patient's perspective
You are Rose Smith, a 50-year-old widow who was diagnosed with leukaemia 1 year ago. You have been seeing the local cancer specialist at the hospital and you have been responding well to treatment. A few days ago you noticed your throat felt quite sore and you had a dry, annoying cough. You are naturally a somewhat anxious person and are quite worried about these symptoms.

Your suspicion is that the sore throat is a sign that the cancer has come back. You think some antibiotics might help. Your concern is that you want this sore throat cured quickly so the cancer does not get a chance to take hold again.

You are quite anxious and just really want the doctor to decide what is best for you. Equally, you would quite like to know what this sore throat is and be reassured that it is nothing sinister.

- The patient has a concern or expectation about his or her condition or treatment which needs to be elicited.
- The patient wants more information about his or her condition or treatment. Inherent within this is that the patient has a preference for how s/he would like this information presented (e.g. using pictures, numbers or text).
- The patient has a preference for role involvement in decision-making (paternalistic, shared or consumerist) which needs to be elicited.

It should be noted that there is no one right way to handle these consultations. It is the process that is important, not the outcome. If done well, at the end of the consultation the patient role-player should feel more informed and more able to manage the condition. The 'patient' should also feel quite satisfied with the consultation process: that his or

---

Box 6.4 Practice nurse–patient role-play example

Practice nurse's perspective (Ms Evans)

One of your roles in the practice is to monitor regularly the blood pressure of patients diagnosed with hypertension. Today you are seeing John White, a 45-year-old man who was diagnosed with hypertension 6 months ago. From the notes, you discover that his father died of a heart attack at age 52. Mr White's blood pressure reading is high, at 180/115 mmHg. His current medication is a beta-blocker for the control of his hypertension and he injects insulin for his diabetes, diagnosed some years ago.

Mr White is well known to the practice and is a friendly and easy-going fellow. You suspect that he is not taking his tablets and probably has not followed your previous advice about decreasing the amount of salt and fat in his diet. Mr White tells you he is a smoker.

You would like to help Mr White understand the importance of changing his lifestyle and taking his tablets.

Patient perspective (John White)

You are a 45-year-old works foreman. You were diagnosed with diabetes several years ago and you regularly inject insulin. Six months ago you were diagnosed with high blood pressure, for which the doctor gave you some tablets.

You have never found compliance with dietary advice or medication easy and would readily admit as much. Your philosophy is, 'If it's a toss-up between behaving myself and living a life, I'd rather live a life.' Although your dad died of a heart attack at age 52, you remember him fondly as a man who had many friends with whom he shared the odd pint.

When you have taken your tablets, you have experienced giddiness and faintness. This is quite a concern for you because you need to keep your wits about you while at work where you are surrounded by heavy machinery. If asked, you would describe yourself as a social smoker – around 20 cigarettes a day.

You would quite like to know more about high blood pressure and what your options are. At the moment you are not too inclined to make any radical changes to your lifestyle.

If the nurse asks if you would like to be involved in the process of deciding how best to manage your blood pressure, you should be amenable, if a little unsure about exactly what she might mean. You could mention that you'd quite like to 'have a say' in deciding what is the best way forward for you.

---

her concerns have been 'listened to' and acknowledged by the 'health-care professional'.

Boxes 6.2–6.4 provide uniprofessional role-plays for learners to try out their concordance skills. It is intended that these role-plays provide a relevant context for practising concordance skills for the different healthcare professionals. However, the underlying skills, knowledge and attitudes that need to be employed to enact a concordant consultation successfully are common to all three professional groups. While a multiprofessional role-play involving nurses, doctors and pharmacists with one patient could be devised, such a situation would not reflect the true practice of concordance. It could be argued that should a patient have a concordant consultation with a GP or practice nurse, that patient would not need a subsequent concordant consultation with the pharmacist as his or her concerns and expectations would have been addressed and a mutually agreed action plan already negotiated. However, a subsequent consultation with the pharmacist could reinforce the approach taken by the nurse or physician and may be used to address previously unidentified postconsultation concerns.

However, there are other role-play techniques outwith the fishbowl and multiple approaches. Role reversal can be used to gain insight into the experience of a different perspective with, for example, the person playing the role of the healthcare professional playing the role of patient. Role rotation, where the lead role (the role under scrutiny) moves from one participant to the next, can be used in order to deflect attention from one particular individual while enabling a larger numbers of participants to have the experience of playing the lead role. In addition to these techniques, Van Ments (1989) has described other variations on the role-play technique:

1. Alter ego – a participant (the alter ego) stands behind the role-player and voices the perceived thoughts or feelings of the lead role-player, using first-person statements such as 'I was hurt by the comment.' The alter ego must be sensitive enough to provide feedback without undermining the confidence of the role-player.
2. Supporter – used when the role-player dries up or when the role-play is not going well. The supporter also stands behind the role-player and uses the first-person voice. They can guide the role-player, fill in gaps or may suggest a new direction for the session.
3. Replay – this technique can be used to provide rehearsal, confidence and positive feedback. This is particularly useful with shorter, less elaborate role-plays, where participants can repeat them, or parts of them. 'Pause' can be used to point out a vital feature of the communication process.
4. Consultant group – the role-player protagonist has a home support group to advise him or her on how to proceed. Prior to the role-play, the protagonist meets with the group and discusses how the role-play should be handled. During the role-play there are periodic breaks (time-outs) for the role-player to consult with their group on the best way forward.

5.   Fast-forward – if the role-play is not progressing, the facilitator calls out 'cut' and asks the group to assume that x and y have now happened and to proceed from there. This requires participants who are very comfortable with the technique, but variations on 'replay', 'pause' and 'fast-forward' can be extremely useful if they are used skilfully.

As described by Elwyn *et al.* (2001), these techniques are essentially a means to enable participants to explore roles in more depth and from different angles. Modifications of the role-play technique have been used to improve participants' self-efficacy and outcome expectancies (Parle *et al.*, 1997). Parle and colleagues define self-efficacy as an individual's assessment of his or her ability to perform a specified task successfully. Outcome expectancies are the person's beliefs about the anticipated consequences of the task. Techniques such as pausing the role-play are used to build up a participant's perceived levels of self-efficacy and outcome expectancy. In this context, the lead role-players are asked how they feel at key junctures throughout the role-play; their thoughts and beliefs are explored. A participant is then able to improve those skills that they might find difficult (Parle *et al.*, 1997).

Kurtz *et al.* (1998) advocate using role-play to explore difficult cases participants have experienced in their work. Learners can also be asked to develop their own problem scenarios to demonstrate the specific problem or area of skill development. This technique was further developed by Rollnick *et al.* (2002) as part of their context-bound communication skills training. These participants had their reported difficult cases transformed into scenarios using standardised simulated patients who visited them at their practice base before and after briefing seminars. From the transcripts of these consultations, participants were able to reflect on what they would have liked to have done differently and what key skills they would like to employ when the consultation is repeated. The participant then received another visit from the simulated patient and this process was repeated (Rollnick *et al.*, 2002). This technique is particularly useful for professionals already in practice where the link between key skills and relevance to practice is made explicit. However, this method is both resource- and time-intensive should it need to be replicated for a large number of practitioners. Ultimately, the choice of how an individual training programme will be delivered will be constrained by the time and resources available.

In summary, a range of approaches have been described, including the place of didactic approaches, small-group techniques, the use of role-play with feedback, 'trigger' tapes and narrative. Maguire and Pitceathly

(2002) describe five effective teaching methods for doctors to enable the acquisition of the relevant communication skills and stop using blocking behaviour:

1. Provide evidence of current deficiencies in communication, reasons for them, and the consequences for doctors and patients.
2. Offer an evidence base for the skills needed to overcome these deficiencies.
3. Demonstrate the skills to be learned and elicit reactions for these.
4. Provide an opportunity to practise the skills under controlled and safe conditions.
5. Give constructive feedback on performance and reflect on the reasons for any blocking behaviour.

This list provides the foundation on which concordance training should be based, reinforcing the need for a range of quite specific teaching methods to facilitate student learning.

Structure of the training

There are no immutable rules about the structure of a training programme in concordance. There is no one method which has been shown to deliver the optimal skill base, be most acceptable to participants, achieve the most favourable change in subsequent professional behaviour or improve patient health status outcomes. The recent Cochrane review identified 17 research studies involving interventions for health-care professionals that sought to promote a patient-centred approach in clinical consultations (Lewin *et al.*, 2002). In these 17 studies, a range of approaches were used, from one highly structured 30-minute private interview with a programme director (Cope *et al.*, 1986) to 22.5 hours of specific communication training over a 6-month period (Langewitz *et al.*, 1998). None the less, there are goals or ideals which should underpin the structure of any training programme. These three core structural attributes are that the training should be:

- recurring
- integrated
- relevant to practice

Firstly, learning in concordance is not a one-off event but one that is developed, supported and reinforced throughout one's professional career. Concordance, as part of lifelong learning, is not a group of skills that can be mastered and set aside. Rather it is part of an approach to practice that will continually be challenged and re-evaluated throughout one's professional career. Secondly, concordance training should be integrated with other learning, not quarantined from it. In this sense concordance training should be seen as a vertical theme throughout training. This is particularly important at an undergraduate level where concordance skill development should be seen as integral to basic clinical training, sociology teaching, ethics courses or practice-based attachments. Kurtz *et al.* (1998) identify several strategies for integrating communication skills with clinical training. These strategies include dividing skills into segments which can be offered at intervals, devising a summary of skills which conveys to other course directors the core content of the training and the use of communication skills to solve patient problems. Integration is best facilitated through the use of a consistent framework for teaching and evaluating skills (Laidlaw *et al.*, 2002).

Finally, as explained by Rollnick *et al.* (2002), a contextualised workshop which provides learning experiences closely related to professionals' working lives, is particularly appropriate for more established learners. In Rollnick *et al.* (2002), the workshop training took place at the GP's workplace, was directed by the everyday concerns of physicians and focused on their management of a simulated consultation conducted during routine clinical work. Relevance to practice is important at all levels of training. However, as the skills and experience of a learner increase, it is particularly important for the content of the training to be driven by the needs of the workplace. Further, the method of training should closely resemble the workplace environment. Using a hypothetical role-play in a university environment may be appropriate for undergraduates learning new skills; a role-play enacted in the workplace driven by problems identified in the workplace is more appropriate for more experienced learners.

How will it be assessed?

Assessment is a complex issue and has been the subject of much recent commentary and debate. The purpose of this section is not to review this vast literature, nor is it to be prescriptive and propose one ideal method of assessment suitable for training in concordance. Rather, its purpose is to raise some important issues to consider when designing an appropriate assessment method and, in particular, to focus on two specific issues of relevance to concordance training: the use of feedback and rating scales.

There are two purposes of assessment: summative and formative. Summative assessment is an end-of-course assessment that includes a measure that sums up a person's achievement. Summative assessment provides 'feedout', in the form of a warrant to achievement or competence (such as a degree certificate) (Knight, 2001). Such assessments should be matched to the learning objectives of the course and should reflect the goals and philosophy of the course (Kurtz *et al.*, 1998: 171). The purpose of formative assessment is to get an estimate of achievement which is used to help in the learning process (Brown and Knight, 1994). Formative assessment might include coursework where learners receive feedback that helps them to improve their next performance or may include discussion between a mentor and a learner. Formative assessment works best when it relates to clear criteria and where the comments are not accompanied by marks or grades (Black, 1998). Both summative and formative assessment may share the same method, such as a checklist or rating scale for judging role-play performance.

There is a broad range of assessment techniques. Knight (2001) outlines 50 assessment methods, from computer-based self-assessment to short appraisals of target papers to games or simulations. Learner self-assessment, peer assessment and group assessment are other techniques which can add diversity to the range of assessment approaches and formats (Race, 2001). Brown (1999) argues that, in designing an assessment, we should use an assessment method which is 'fit for purpose' by asking ourselves the following questions:

- Why are we assessing?
- What are we assessing?
- How are we assessing?
- Who is best placed to assess?
- When should we assess?

In this sense, the methods of assessment should mirror the methods of instruction. As suggested by Kurtz *et al.* (1998), the method of assessment should encourage learners to work and study for summative assessments using the methods of learning employed in the training programme itself. One such approach is an objective, structured clinical evaluation (OSCE). In an OSCE, a learner is assessed by direct observation of his or her ability to communicate with simulated patients in a standardised evaluation setting that is as close as possible to true life (Kurtz *et al.*, 1998). This is a form of summative assessment which allows for the integration of concordance communication skills with clinical skills and suitably mirrors the skills-based teaching of role-play.

Increasingly used as part of certifying examinations for physicians in the USA and Canada, and more recently in the UK (Southgate *et al.*, 2001), considerable research has been undertaken on the validity and reliability of the OSCE (Van der Vleuten and Swanson, 1990; Vu and Barrows, 1994; Cusimano, 1996; Kaufman *et al.*, 2000).

Feedback

The mainstay of experiential learning using role-plays is the use of observation and feedback. As discussed by Rogers (2001), feedback should offer description, not opinion. Feedback can be provided in the small-group setting or as part of one-to-one teaching. As noted by Kurtz *et al.* (1998: 43), 'feedback needs to be specific, detailed, non-judgemental and well-intentioned'. Rogers (2001) makes several distinctions between feedback and criticism (Table 6.2). Although these are obvious points – particularly for more experienced learners – they are points worth reiterating before the role-play begins.

Following observation of the role-play, the traditional approach to feedback has been to draw upon the method or 'rules' of Pendleton *et al.* (1984). Pendleton's rules exhort learners and facilitators to state positive issues first, to give the learner the opportunity to comment first and for observers to be constructive in their comments, suggesting how improvements to the interaction could be made.

Table 6.2   Differences between feedback and criticism

Feedback	*Criticism*
Designed to improve performance positively	A way of unloading anger and disappointment
Calm	Angry, tart, dismissive, emotional
Tough on the performance	Tough on the person
Specific – describes the facts	Vague, generalised, uses words like 'you always' or 'you never'
Focuses on the future; makes suggestions about positive alternatives	Looks backwards
Two-way – solicits the learner's opinions	One-way

Adapted from Rogers (2001) with permission.

However, there are difficulties associated with the rigid adherence to the Pendleton rules (Kurtz *et al.*, 1998). In a feedback session, it may be artificial to separate good points from bad points and, given the limitations of time, too long may be spent on discussing good points and/or in not probing issues of importance to the learner. To overcome some of these potential difficulties, Silverman *et al.* (1996) have outlined the agenda-led, outcome-based analysis for providing feedback. Key features of this approach are shown in Box 6.5.

Further information on this approach, including greater detail on how to run a session using this feedback method, is provided in chapter 5 of Kurtz *et al.* (1998). The agenda-led, outcome-based analysis is an approach which lends itself to concordance training although, to get the most out of the session, it may demand greater facilitation skills than the traditional Pendleton approach.

Rating scales and checklists

Boon and Stewart (1998) reviewed the instruments to assess patient–physician interactions that were available between 1986 and 1996. They identified 16 communication assessment tools used in education. These tools included those which involved real-time assessment

---

Box 6.5   Principles of agenda-led, outcome-based analysis for providing feedback

- Start with the learner's agenda
- Look at the outcomes the learner and patient are trying to achieve
- Encourage self-assessment and self problem-solving first
- Involve the whole group in problem-solving
- Use descriptive feedback to encourage a non-judgemental approach
- Provide balanced feedback
- Make offers and suggestions; generate alternatives
- Rehearse suggestions by 'replaying' the role-play
- Be well-intentioned, valuing and supportive
- Value the interaction as a gift of raw material for the group
- Opportunistically introduce concepts, principles, research evidence and wider discussion
- Structure and summarise learning so that a constructive end-point is reached

Adapted from Kurtz *et al.* (1998) with permission.

by an observer, an assessment by the trained patient-actor involved in the interaction, assessment by an observer using a video- or audiotape of the interaction and those which used self-report, by either the patient or the physician. The tools used could be rating scales (e.g. with '1' representing 'poor' and '5' representing 'excellent'), checklists or interactional analyses. In the review Boon and Stewart (1998) conclude that few of the instruments have been used widely, many have never been demonstrated to be reliable or valid and few have been compared with each other. It should be noted that these assessment tools focus on the process of the interaction rather than on patient outcomes such as satisfaction, adherence to medication, recall and understanding of information or health status/psychiatric morbidity (Ong *et al.*, 1995). With more experienced learners, such as those undertaking concordance training as part of continuing professional development, the use of patient-based assessments which provide feedback on the professional's interpersonal skills becomes increasingly relevant and important. Although commonly used as part of research, patient-based assessments have been less frequently used for educational purposes (Boon and Stewart, 1998). A questionnaire evaluating doctors' interpersonal skills which incorporates both the educational and patient perspectives has recently been described (Greco *et al.*, 2000) and validated (Greco *et al.*, 1999).

Two instruments may be particularly useful in relation to training and education in concordance. Both contain items which relate to the four aims or domains described in Table 6.1 (page 98). The SEGUE framework is a 25- or 32-item checklist that employs a nominal (yes/no) scale (Makoul *et al.*, 1995; Makoul, 2001). The five sections of the SEGUE framework include: (1) setting the stage; (2) eliciting information; (3) giving information; (4) understanding the patient's perspective; and (5) ending the encounter. The most recent work provides greater detail on the validity and reliability of this tool (Makoul, 2001).

The second instrument is the Calgary-Cambridge Observation Guide (Kurtz *et al.*, 1998). This uses a five-point plan within which the individual skills are structured. These five areas are: (1) initiating the session; (2) gathering information; (3) building the relationship; (4) explanation and planning; and (5) closing the session. The guides are provided in two sections. Guide One focuses on interviewing the patient and contains 33 items. Guide Two concerns explanation and planning and contains up to 40 items, depending upon the content of the interaction. The guides use descriptive feedback and are suited to formative assessment or adapted as part of an OSCE. Further details of these guides are provided in Kurtz *et al.* (1998).

Conclusion

This chapter has attempted to identify some of the key issues relevant to the teaching and learning of concordance. Given the evolving nature of the concept of concordance, the intention has not been to be prescriptive in either approach or content. While training in concordance involves communication skill development, it is also much more than that. Concordance necessitates realignment in how we relate to patients, an explicit recognition of the importance of the patient's view and a conviction that, for those patients with concerns, concordance is an appropriate way forward. While concordance has emphasised the importance of the patient perspective, the training issues discussed here also recognise the importance of the professional in a learning role. Concordance calls for a reflective professional, one who is aware of the influence of his or her own personal values on the nature of his or her relationships with patients. This professional takes the time to identify his or her own learning needs and to engage in training actively, implicitly recognising the importance of learning by doing. The use of specific techniques such as role-play are an attempt to mirror professional practice in order to underline the fundamental relationship between active learning, reflective practice and continuing professional development.

References

Black P (1998). Learning, league tables and national assessment. *Oxford Rev Educ* 24: 57–68.

Boon H, Stewart M (1998). Patient–physician communication assessment instruments: 1986–1996 in review. *Patient Educ Couns* 35: 161–176.

Branch W T, Kern D, Haidet P *et al.* (2001). Teaching the human dimensions of care in clinical settings. *JAMA* 286: 1067–1074.

Britten N, Stevenson F A, Barry C A *et al.* (2000). Misunderstandings in prescribing decisions in general practice: qualitative study. *BMJ* 320: 484–488.

Brown S (1999). Institutional strategies for assessment. In: Brown S, Glasner A (eds) *Assessment Matters in Higher Education – Choosing and Using Diverse Approaches*. Buckingham: Society for Research into Higher Education and Open University Press, 3–13.

Brown S, Knight P (1994). *Assessing Learners in Higher Education*. London: Kogan Page.

Caris-Verhallen W M, Kerkstra A, Bensing J M, Grypdonck M (2000). Effects of video interaction analysis training on nurse–patient communication in the care of the elderly. *Patient Educ Couns* 39: 91–103.

Centre for Pharmacy Postgraduate Education (2002). *'Let's Talk it Through': A Structured Approach to Significant Stories of Medicines Usage – Evaluation Report*. London: HMSO.

Charles C, Gafni A, Whelan T (1999). Decision-making in the physician–patient encounter: revisiting the shared treatment decision-making model. *Soc Sci Med* 49: 651–661.

Cope D W, Linn L S, Leake B D, Barrett P A (1986). Modification of residents' behavior by preceptor feedback of patient satisfaction. *J Gen Intern Med* 1: 394–398.

Coté L, Leclere H (2000). How clinical teachers perceive the doctor–patient relationship and themselves as role models. *Acad Med* 75:1117–1124.

Cusimano M (1996). Standard-setting in medical education. *Acad Med* 71(suppl. 10): S112–S120.

Davis D A, Thomson M A, Oxman A D, Haynes R B (1995). Changing physician performance – a systematic review of the effect of continuing medical education strategies. *JAMA* 274: 700–705.

Denicolo P, Entwistle N, Hounsell D (1992). *What is Active Learning? Effective Learning and Teaching in Higher Education Module 1.* Sheffield: CVCP Universities' Staff Development and Training Unit.

DiBartola L M (2001). Listening to patients and responding with care: a model for teaching communication skills. *Joint Commission J Qual Improve* 27: 315–323.

Edwards A, Elwyn G (2001). *Evidence-Based Patient Choice – Inevitable or Impossible?* Oxford: Oxford University Press.

Elwyn G, Greenhalgh T, Macfarlane F (2001). *Groups – A Guide to Small Group Work in Healthcare, Management, Education and Research.* Abingdon: Radcliffe Medical Press.

Elwyn G, Edwards A, Kinnersley P, Grol R (2000). Shared decision-making and the concept of equipoise: defining the competences of involving patients in healthcare choices. *Br J Gen Pract* 50: 892–899.

Greco M, Cavanagh M, Brownlea A, McGovern J (1999). The doctors' interpersonal skills questionnaire (DISQ): a validated instrument for use in GP training. *Educ Gen Pract* 10: 256–264.

Greco M, Brownlea A, McGovern J, Cavanagh M (2000). Consumers as educators: implementation of patient feedback in general practice training. *Health Commun* 12: 173–193.

Greenhalgh T (2001). Storytelling should be targeted where it is known to have greatest added value. *Med Educ* 35: 818.

Greenhalgh T, Hurwitz B (1999). Narrative based medicine – why study narrative? *BMJ* 318: 48–50.

Hargie O D W, Morrow N C, Woodman C (2000). Pharmacists' evaluation of key communication skills in practice. *Patient Educ Couns* 39: 61–70.

James D, Nastasic S, Horne R, Davis G (2001). The design and evaluation of a simulated-patient teaching programme to develop the consultation skills of undergraduate pharmacy students. *Pharm World Sci* 23: 212–216.

Kaufman D M (2003). Applying educational theory in practice. *BMJ* 326: 213–216.

Kaufman D M, Mann K V, Muijtjens A M, Van der Vleuten C P M (2000). A comparison of standard-setting procedures for an OSCE in undergraduate medical education. *Acad Med* 75: 267–271.

Kinmonth A-L, Spiegal N, Woodcock A (1996). Developing a training programme in patient-centred consulting for evaluation in a randomised controlled trial;

diabetes care from diagnosis in British primary care. *Patient Educ Couns* 29: 75–86.

Knight P (2001). *A Briefing on Key Concepts – Formative and Summative, Criterion and Norm-Referenced Assessment*. Assessment series no. 7. York: Learning and Teaching Support Network Generic Centre.

Knowles M S (1980). *The Modern Practice of Adult Education: From Pedagogy to Andragogy*. New York: Adult Education Company.

Kruijver I P M, Kerkstra A, Francke A L *et al.* (2000). Evaluation of communication training programs in nursing care: a review of the literature. *Patient Educ Couns* 39: 129–145.

Kurtz S, Silverman J, Draper J (1998). *Teaching and Learning Communication Skills in Medicine*. Abingdon: Radcliffe Medical Press.

Laidlaw T S, MacLeod H, Kaufman D M *et al.* (2002). Implementing a communication skills programme in medical school: needs assessment and programme change. *Med Educ* 36: 115–124.

Langewitz W A, Eich P, Kiss A, Wossmer B (1998). Improving communication skills – a randomised controlled behaviorally oriented intervention study for residents in internal medicine. *Psychosom Med* 60: 268–276.

Launer J (2002). *Narrative-Based Primary Care – A Practical Guide*. Oxford: Radcliffe Medical Press.

Lewin S A, Skea Z C, Entwistle V *et al.* (2002). *Interventions for Providers to Promote a Patient-Centred Approach in Clinical Consultations* (Cochrane review). The Cochrane Library, issue 4. Oxford: Update Software.

Maguire P, Pitceathly C (2002). Key communication skills and how to acquire them. *BMJ* 325: 697–700.

Makoul G (2001). The SEGUE framework for teaching and assessing communication skills. *Patient Educ Couns* 45: 23–34.

Makoul G, Arntson P, Schofield T (1995). Health promotion in primary care: physician–patient communication and decision-making about prescription medications. *Soc Sci Med* 41: 1241–1254.

Marinker M (2000). Achieving concordance. *Primary Care Pharm* 1: 93–95. Available online at: www.pharmj.com/PrimaryCarePharmacy/200009/comment/viewpoint_concordance.html (accessed 5 April 2004).

Marvel K M, Epstein R M, Flower K, Beckman H B (1999). Soliciting the patient's agenda – have we improved? *JAMA* 281: 283–287.

Mead N, Bower P (2000). Patient-centredness: a conceptual framework and review of the empirical literature. *Soc Sci Med* 51: 1087–1110.

Novack D H, Suchman A L, Clark W *et al.* (1997). Calibrating the physician – personal awareness and effective patient care. *JAMA* 278: 502–509.

Ong L M L, de Haes J, Hoos A M, Lammes F B (1995). Doctor–patient communication: a review of the literature. *Soc Sci Med* 40: 903–918.

Parle M, Maguire P, Heaven C (1997). The development of a training model to improve health professionals' skills, self-efficacy and outcome expectancies when communicating with cancer patients. *Soc Sci Med* 44: 231–240.

Pendleton D, Schofield T, Tate P *et al.* (1984). *The Consultation: An Approach to Learning and Teaching*. Oxford: Oxford University Press.

Race P (2001). *A Briefing on Self, Peer and Group Assessment*. Assessment series no. 9. York: Learning and Teaching Support Network Generic Centre.

Revans R W (1982). *The Origins and Growth of Action Learning*. Bromley, Kent: Chartwell-Brant.

Rogers J (2001). *Adults Learning*, 4th edn. Buckingham: Open University Press.

Rollnick S, Kinnersley P, Butler C (2002). Context-bound communication skills training: development of a new method. *Med Educ* 36: 377–383.

Roter D L, Hall J A, Kern D E *et al.* (1995). Improving physicians' interviewing skills and reducing patients' emotional distress. *Arch Intern Med* 155: 1877–1884.

Silverman J D, Kurtz S M, Draper J (1996). The Calgary-Cambridge approach to communication skills teaching. 1. Agenda-led, outcome-based analysis of the consultation. *Educ Gen Pract* 7: 288–299.

Smith R C, Marshall-Dorsey A A, Osborn G G *et al.* (2000). Evidence-based guidelines for teaching patient-centred interviewing. *Patient Educ Couns* 39: 27–36.

Southgate L, Campbell M, Cox J *et al.* (2001). The General Medical Council's performance procedures: the development and implementation of tests of competence with examples from general practice. *Med Educ* 35 (suppl. 1): 20–28.

Stewart M (1995). Effective physician–patient communication and health outcomes: a review. *Can Med Assoc J*. 152: 1423–1433.

Thomson O'Brien M A, Freemantle N, Oxman A D *et al.* (2004). *Continuing Education Meetings and Workshops: Effects on Professional Practice and Health Care Outcomes* (Cochrane review). The Cochrane Library, issue 4. Oxford: Update Software.

Tiberius R G (1999). *Small Group Teaching – A Troubleshooting Guide*. London: Kogan Page.

Towle A, Godolphin W (1999). Framework for teaching and learning informed shared decision making. *BMJ* 319: 766–771.

Van der Vleuten C P M, Swanson D B (1990). Assessment of clinical skills with standardized patients: state of the art. *Teach Learn Med* 2: 58–76.

Van Ments M (1989). *The Effective Use of Role-Play*. London: Kogan Page.

Vu N V, Barrows H (1994). Use of standardised patients in clinical assessments: recent developments and measurement findings. *Educ Res* 23: 23–50.

Watson M C, Bond C M, Grimshaw J M *et al.* (2002). Educational strategies to promote evidence-based community pharmacy practice: a cluster randomized controlled trial (RCT). *Fam Pract* 19: 529–536.

Wilkinson S (1991). Factors which influence how nurses communicate with cancer patients. *J Adv Nurs* 16: 677–688.

7

The theoretical basis of concordance and issues for research

Robert Horne and John Weinman

Introduction

The aim of this chapter is to present a research perspective on the concept of concordance. We will begin by identifying key questions about concordance and its potential impact on healthcare. We will then present a research strategy for addressing some of the questions that arise from the concept of concordance.

What is concordance and how can we recognise it?

Before we can systematically evaluate the value of concordance we need to define clearly what we mean by concordance. Only then can we begin to *operationalise* the concept, to decide how it can be recognised and measured. Concordance is a difficult concept to define exactly but few would disagree with its central tenet that prescribing should take account of patients' beliefs and expectations and involve patients as partners in their own healthcare. However, in its original form the concept appears to go further, as shown by this definition from the Concordance website:

> Concordance is a new approach to the prescribing and taking of medicines. It is an agreement reached after negotiation between a patient and a health care professional that respects the beliefs and wishes of the patient in determining whether, when and how medicines are to be taken. Although reciprocal, this is an alliance in which the health care professionals recognise the primacy of the patient's decisions about taking the recommended medications (www.concordance.org : accessed 27 June 2001).

If we take this definition at face value then the most important attribute of the concordant prescription is one in which the patient's decision has prevailed. If we were to accept this, then we could operationalise concordance on the basis of whether the prescription had reflected 'the primacy of the patient's decisions'. Unfortunately, our task is not that simple. If concordance research is to be relevant to policy and practice in healthcare we need to consider its practical implications. The above definition of concordance raises questions about the rights and responsibilities of the individual, which need to be addressed before we can be clear about what we are researching and how we should do it.

How does concordance relate to notions of 'rights and responsibilities'?

It may be too simplistic to consider the consultation in isolation. It is more than a meeting between patient and clinician (we have used the generic term 'clinician' to indicate doctor, pharmacist, nurse or other healthcare professional). The core decision involves at least three parties: the patient, the prescriber and the payer. A philosophy of prescribing which ignores the payer may be noble but ultimately is limited in its capacity to foster pragmatic solutions to questions of how best to use medicines. Within the UK NHS, the prescriber is responsible for allocating resources on behalf of society and the needs of the individual must be viewed in the context of the needs of others. What happens when the patient's preferences conflict with the 'greater good'? Let us consider a patient whose wish is to be prescribed an expensive new medicine but the prevailing evidence suggests that the medicine will not be effective. The prescriber expresses this belief to the patient with an explanation of the rationale for not prescribing the medicine. The patient remains unconvinced and reiterates his or her decision that s/he wants the clinician to prescribe the medicine. A key question here is how advocates of the concept of concordance would advise the clinician to proceed. Should the clinician accept the 'predominance of the patient's decision', as implied within the above definition, and prescribe the medicine to attain concordance? Or should s/he refuse to prescribe on the grounds that, based on the available evidence, the prescription would divert healthcare resources from cases where the benefits are clearer? Thus a simple interpretation of the assertion within the concordance philosophy that the patient's decision or views predominate may be difficult to justify from a utilitarian perspective, reducing its application within the NHS. Similarly, the patient's decision could not be justified from an evidence-based perspective.

How does concordance relate to evidence-based medicine?

The hypothetical example described above illustrates the potential tension between two of the prevailing ideas in the debate about the future of medicine: evidence-based medicine and patient-centred medicine. What happens when the patient's preferences conflict with the prevailing evidence? What if a patient rejects a potentially life-saving treatment (such as immunosuppressant therapy following renal transplantation) due to erroneous interpretations of the likely risks vs. benefits or because of beliefs that are factually incorrect? A similar set of questions apply in circumstances where the patient's preferences could result in harm to the patient or others.

For many illnesses and treatments, the relationship between taking medication and outcome is unclear. However, in others, the evidence is much stronger. In such cases it is inappropriate to advocate the primacy of the patient's decision if this is based on erroneous beliefs. Here the duty of the clinician is to promote informed choice. In cases where patients' choices are informed by erroneous interpretations of the prevailing evidence (e.g. the likely risks and benefits of treatment) or on misplaced beliefs, then passively 'respecting' these beliefs or 'agreeing to differ' might represent a lapse in care and duty to the patient. A more active approach is warranted where the clinician tries to identify and alter misconceptions and to challenge beliefs that appear to be incompatible with the prevailing evidence.

These issues are relevant to the research agenda. For proponents of concordance there is an underlying assumption that concordance is the best approach, but as researchers we must be aware of all the possible outcomes and try to be objective in the way we identify and measure them.

From concordance to adherence: a step backwards or the way forward?

Until the intellectual foundation of the concept of concordance is more firmly established it is difficult to define a specific research agenda. More work is needed to clarify these concepts and how they relate to the ethics of prescribing, communication about medicines and medicines-taking. As other chapters in this book illustrate, this work is progressing. However, in the interim, we believe that there is an imperative to research better ways of helping patients to get the most from their medicines.

To do this we may need to move back a little along the road from compliance to concordance. If we are to understand and optimise the use of medicines, we need to assess what people actually do with medicines and the degree to which this matches the recommendations. We cannot ignore the fact that medicines and most other treatments need to be used in a particular way if they are to be effective and safe. A fundamental part of this research agenda will be considerations of adherence (the extent to which the patient's behaviour matches the clinician's recommendation).

One unfortunate outcome of the concordance initiative is that the term 'concordance' is now often used as a synonym for compliance or adherence (e.g. 'The intervention was designed to improve patient concordance'). This is not just a problem of semantics. The terms 'adherence' and 'compliance' reflect different perspectives of the same phenomenon: the degree to which the patient's behaviour matches medical advice: for many purposes the terms are interchangeable. These terms describe the behaviour of one individual: the patient. Concordance is a much more complex and less well-defined term relating to the process (e.g. partnership?) and outcomes (agreement or shared decision-making?) of prescribing. A clear prerequisite for a sensible research agenda is to be clear about terminology. It is nonsensical to use the term 'concordance' when we mean 'compliance' or 'adherence'. To do so is a triumph of political correctness over common sense.

The problem is that the term 'compliance' has become associated with an inappropriate, paternalistic model of healthcare in which the patient is expected to follow the doctor's orders. (This may also be true of the term 'adherence'.) However, we still need a method to describe the extent to which the patient's behaviour matches the advice or recommendations of the prescriber. We therefore recommend that the terms 'compliance' or 'adherence' should be used in a value-free way to describe the degree to which behaviour matches recommendations. The concept of good and bad compliance/adherence clearly has no place but referring to high or low compliance/adherence is perfectly acceptable. Although we believe that the terms 'compliance' and 'adherence' may be interchangeable if we define them as above, we will use 'adherence' in the remainder of this chapter. We use 'adherence' to emphasise that it is the patient's right to choose whether or not to follow the doctor's recommendations and that failure to do so should not be a reason for blame.

The concept of informed adherence

The concept of concordance grew from a review of the literature on treatment compliance and discussions within a committee of healthcare researchers, clinicians and managers, established by the Royal Pharmaceutical Society of Great Britain and funded by Merck Sharpe & Dohme (Royal Pharmaceutical Society of Great Britain, 1997). This recognised the importance of patients' personal beliefs about their illness and treatment. Research had shown that patients' perceptions were often at odds with the medical view yet strongly influenced their decision about whether or not to take medication. Non-adherence was often the outcome of a prescribing process that failed to take account of the patient's beliefs, expectations and preferences (McGavock, 1996; Horne, 1998). It could be an indicator of poor communication within the consultation. Moreover, the fault line within the consultation was the failure to recognise that patients and clinicians bring two sets of (potentially opposing) beliefs about the nature of the illness and treatment. Consultations that ignored the patient's perspective would be more likely to lead to treatment decisions that were not 'agreed' by the patient, with an increased risk of non-adherence.

The key contribution of concordance to the debate about the problem of non-adherence is to reinforce the importance of patients' beliefs as one of the determinants of adherence and to identify the consultation as the main source and potential remedy of the problem. At a time when public trust in doctors and science is undoubtedly diminishing (Horton, 2003), a better understanding of patients' beliefs and preferences is a priority for research and clinical practice. Clinicians have an ethical imperative to facilitate informed patient choice about whether or not to adhere to recommendations for the use of medicines and other treatments.

Michie and colleagues (2003) have outlined a model for informed choice in healthcare and this is a good starting point for discussion about informed choice in relation to adherence to medicines. They propose that the key components of informed choice are knowledge and beliefs. Patients can be considered to have made an informed choice if they can demonstrate knowledge of relevant information about the screening test or the treatment and then act according to their beliefs. We suggest that in applying this framework to choice about using treatments that are supported by a strong evidence base, the clinician has a duty that goes beyond providing information. Informing should be an active process, which involves more than simply presenting the evidence. It also entails eliciting the patient's beliefs and identifying whether pre-existing beliefs might act as a barrier to an unbiased interpretation of the evidence. If the interpretation of information is influenced by misconceptions about the illness and treatment, then can the choice be truly informed?

We propose the concept of *informed adherence* as a target for consultations in which evidence-based medicine is used to guide initial recommendations for treatment. These are then presented to patients in a way that takes account of their beliefs and preferences and attempts to help patients resolve any incompatibilities between their personal beliefs and the prevailing evidence.

We believe that this approach is not incompatible with the central tenets of concordance in that it places patients' beliefs and preferences at centre stage within the consultation. A fundamental question that can be addressed is the degree to which the patient's (and clinician's) beliefs and preferences match the available evidence. We are still left, of course, with the problem of uncertainty in medicine. In many cases the available evidence will be inconclusive. Here the goal of the informed choice is to facilitate an interpretation of the available evidence that is unencumbered by misconceptions.

Operationalising concordance in the context of informed adherence

We suggested that facilitating informed adherence to evidence-based prescriptions should be the immediate priority for research and practice We also argue that, although the concept of concordance is still in development, the central tenets are relevant to informed adherence. The concept of the clinical consultation as a meeting of two potentially opposing sets of beliefs about the illness and the treatment is fundamental to an understanding of informed adherence. This aspect of the concordance concept can be easily operationalised and researched in a systematic way since at its core is the need to understand patients' perceptions of their illness and treatment, and how these relate to the perceptions of the clinician and to the prevailing evidence.

Until the concept of the concordance has been fully clarified we suggest that concordance may be defined as *the degree of match or mismatch between two sets of beliefs*. This could entail a comparison between the beliefs of the patient and the prescriber (or other, e.g. carer or other healthcare professional) or an assessment of the degree to which the patient's beliefs are consistent with medical evidence. This definition could be used as a basis for operationalising key aspects of the concept that could inform a research agenda even while some of the outstanding questions about the concept, such as those outlined above, are being resolved.

A concordance-related research agenda

Extending the current knowledge base

We already know a lot about adherence. Over the last few decades, numerous research studies have examined the causes of non-adherence and some have tested interventions to improve adherence rates (Haynes *et al.*, 1996). Box 7.1 presents some of the main insights from this research, in order to provide a context for concordance-related research into informed adherence. This research has been summarised in a recent report by the World Health Organization (2003).

One of the most important insights over the last decade has been the recognition of the importance of public beliefs about

---

Box 7.1 An outline of current knowledge about adherence

- It is estimated that over 30% of prescribed medication is not taken as directed
- If the prescription was appropriate then this level of non-adherence represents a significant loss to patients and the healthcare system
- Non-adherence is common across most medical conditions and for most types of treatment
- Sociodemographic or trait personality characteristics do not appear to be strong predictors of adherence; rates vary within individuals across time and different treatments
- Non-adherence may be *unintentional* when patients' intentions to take prescribed medication are thwarted by barriers such as forgetting, poor comprehension or difficulties in opening the packaging or the intentional result of a decision by the patient not take the medication or to take less or more than recommended
- Few interventions to promote adherence have proved effective
- Interventions to facilitate adherence are likely to be more effective if they take account of the causes of intentional and unintentional non-adherence
- Adherence behaviours are often undeclared within the consultation
- Few patients volunteer reports of non-adherence, perhaps because they fear that the prescriber will be disappointed or offended
- Decisions about adherence are influenced by patients' personal beliefs about the illness and treatment
- Patients' beliefs are sometimes based on erroneous information or misconceptions about the illness and the relative benefits and risks of the treatment

pharmaceuticals in determining adherence. The key challenge for research is to develop methods for eliciting adherence-related beliefs and preferences and to help health-providers to take account of these beliefs in the way in which treatments are presented and negotiated. This research will need to move beyond an examination of individual barriers and drivers to adherence. We will also need theoretical models relating patient beliefs and adherence that can be used as a basis for developing and testing complex interventions to facilitate informed adherence. Research should include, but not be limited to, the consultation. It also needs to focus on individuals and factors other than contact with clinicians that might influence medicines usage. Finally, attempts to understand and promote informed adherence should consider macro-level issues such as the relationship between knowledge and beliefs as well as the role of sources of knowledge other than clinicians.

The components of informed adherence

Peoples' use of medicines is influenced by a wide variety of variables and the complex interaction between them. However, we can identify several core factors that need to be addressed if we are to encourage informed adherence. We need to consider the individual's beliefs, knowledge, issues of empowerment/inclusion and skills, and the contextual issues that influence interactions between these factors. Fortunately we are not starting with an empty slate. Recent research has identified some of the key determinants of adherence decisions. This has not only improved our understanding of patient perspectives of medicine-taking but has also led to developments in measurement and theory (Horne, 2003).

Utilising theory in the design of adherence-related interventions is fundamental to our research strategy. Indeed, the use of theory is one of the mainstays of the Medical Research Council's recommendations for the design and testing of complex interventions (Campbell *et al.*, 2000) (www.mrc.ac.uk). Theories guide the selection of targets for change (e.g. the types of beliefs or processes that we need to elicit and address) and allow the assessment of process as well as outcome. This is important if we are to understand why a particular approach has affected or not affected outcome in the way we hypothesised.

A number of theoretical models have been developed to explain health-related behaviour and several of these might be applied to improve our understanding of informed adherence. These models share the common assumption that the motivation to engage in and maintain

health-related behaviours arises from beliefs that influence the interpretation of information and experiences and guide behaviour (see
Horne and Weinman (1998) for an overview of theoretical approaches
to adherence and Conner and Norman (1996) for a more detailed
review of social cognition models).

We have suggested that the concept of concordance hinges on the
degree to which patients' perception of their disease or condition and
their beliefs about treatment correspond to (or are *concordant* with)
those of the clinician and/or the evidence base. It follows that theoretical
models that specify beliefs about illness and treatment as antecedents
of adherence are likely to be particularly relevant. Leventhal's self-
regulatory model (or common-sense model) was developed specifically
to explain how people process information about illness (Leventhal
et al., 1992). It argues that people form 'common-sense' beliefs about
illness that may differ from the medical view yet influence decision
about treatment, including adherence decisions. Recently the model has
been adapted to address medication adherence by considering patients'
'common-sense' ideas about treatment as well as their perceptions of illness (Horne, 1997, 2003). Thus Leventhal's common-sense model offers
a framework that can be used to operationalise the concordance construct and investigate its relevance to informed adherence (Horne and
Weinman, 2002).

Assessing beliefs about illness and processing illness-related information

The self-regulation theory or common-sense model developed by
Howard Leventhal and colleagues (1992) conceptualises the patient as
an 'active problem solver' whose behaviour in response to an illness
(e.g. taking or not taking prescribed medication) reflects an attempt to
manage the illness in a way which makes common sense to him or her.
The model suggests that people are rarely inclined 'blindly' to follow
health advice, even if it is provided by clinicians whom they respect.
Rather, people tend to interpret the advice and make a decision about
whether they should follow it.

When we are faced with a health threat (e.g. experiencing symptoms or being told by a physician that we have a particular disease), our
first response is to form a 'mental map' or 'model' of the condition. This
helps us to 'make sense' of the condition and guides the action we take
to remedy the perceived problem. Patient illness models are referred to
using several terms: illness beliefs, illness perceptions and illness representations. For the purposes of this discussion these terms are

interchangeable as they essentially mean the same thing: patients' personal ideas about their illness. Leventhal suggests that illness perceptions have the following important attributes:

1. Patients' personal ideas about their illness are often organised around five components: identity, timeline, cause, consequences and control/cure. These can be thought of as the answers to five basic questions about the illness or health threat: (1) What is it? (2) How long will it last? (3) What caused it? (4) How will it affect/has it affected me? (5) Can it be controlled or cured? People form a mental model or representation of the illness which is made up of their answers to these questions.
2. Symptom perceptions have a strong influence on patients' ideas about their illness and upon subsequent behaviour. Basically, patients are more likely to perceive their condition as a problem, and try to rectify it, if they associate it with unpleasant symptoms unless they have an alternative model that makes common sense (e.g. prophylaxis or prevention). In other words, the experience of symptoms is fundamental to our thinking about illness. Taking a treatment for a condition which does not appear to have any symptoms may appear to go against 'common sense' unless the patient is provided with a clear rationale for why the treatment is being recommended (e.g. prophylaxis)

Illness perceptions have a direct and logical effect on behaviour and outcomes. For example, if patients believe that their problem was primarily caused by stress, then they will be very likely to avoid or disengage from potentially stressful situations. Patients' own ideas about the illness may have a stronger influence on their behaviour than the advice of healthcare practitioners.

Beliefs about prescribed medication: the necessity–concerns framework

Once we begin to see patients as active problem-solvers it follows that, in deciding whether to adhere to a treatment schedule, the patient has to think not only about whether the illness warrants treatment but also whether the treatment is appropriate for the illness.

Given the importance of medicines in healthcare and the apparently widespread problem of non-adherence, surprisingly little attention has focused on how people perceive and make decisions about medicines. There are a few notable exceptions (see Horne (1997) for a review). Several seminal studies had used qualitative methods to explore people's perceptions of medications (Arluke, 1980; Gabe and Lipshitz Phillips, 1982; Coulter, 1985; Morgan and Watkins, 1988). These reported similarities in people's ideas about medicines (e.g. that medicines are addictive and accumulate within the body to produce 'long-term' effects) that seemed to be common across locations and cultures (USA, UK and Europe) and illness/treatment categories (Horne, 1997). Similar findings have been reported in more recent qualitative studies (see Chapter 3 in this volume), suggesting that research has identified some of the main themes in public perceptions of medicines.

These studies and our own preliminary interviews conducted with people with chronic medical problems (cardiovascular disease and renal impairment) led us to question whether the commonly expressed beliefs about prescribed medicines could be summarised under simple core themes. We therefore began our investigation of medication beliefs by exploring the principal components underlying representations of prescribed medication. These analyses showed that, although patients' ideas about medicines are often complex and diverse, many of the beliefs relating to prescribed medication could be grouped under two categories: perceptions of *necessity* or personal need for the treatment, and *concerns* about negative effects (Horne *et al.*, 1999).

Necessity beliefs

Studies in a range of chronic medical conditions showed that people who were prescribed the same medication for the same condition, differed in their perceptions of personal need for it (necessity beliefs are operationialised by statements such as 'My health depends on this medicine', 'These medicines protect me from becoming worse' and 'Without these medicines I would be very ill') (Horne and Weinman, 1999; Horne *et al.*, 1999). It is worth noting that perceived necessity is not a form of efficacy belief (a belief about whether the treatment will be effective). Although views about efficacy are likely to contribute to perceived need, the constructs are not synonymous. We might believe that a treatment will be effective but yet not perceive a personal *need* for it. In a recent study of beliefs about antiretroviral medication, the belief that it would be effective at controlling HIV progression explained about 25% of the variance in perceived need (Horne *et al.*, 2002). Conversely, we might perceive a strong need for a treatment that we perceive to be only moderately effective, because we know that it is the only treatment that is available. We anticipate that *necessity* beliefs will be more closely related to adherence than beliefs about treatment efficacy.

Concerns about medication

Studies of patients prescribed different types of medication for a range of illnesses show a similarity in the type of concerns that patients report about prescription medicines. These include concerns about the concrete experiences of unpleasant symptoms as medication 'side-effects' and the disruptive effects of medication on daily living, as well as more abstract worries that regular use could lead to dependence or that the medication would accumulate within the body and lead to obscure, long-term effects. These core concerns seem to be fairly generic and relevant across a range of disease states and cultures, and they are typically endorsed by over a third of study participants (Horne and Weinman, 2002; Horne *et al.*, 1999, 2001a, 2004; Webb *et al.*, 2001). Other concerns are specific to the particular class of medicine (Horne, 2003), for example, worries that corticosteroid inhalers prescribed for asthma will result in weight gain (Hand and Bradley, 1996) or that regular use of analgesic medication now will make it less effective in the future (Gill and Williams, 2001).

Studies involving patients from several illness groups (including asthma, diabetes, kidney disease, heart disease and cancer) have shown that necessity beliefs and concerns are related to reported adherence. Patients with stronger beliefs in the necessity of their medication were more adherent: those with stronger concerns were less adherent (Horne and Weinman, 1999). The negative correlation between concerns and reported adherence suggests that patients may respond to fears about potential adverse effects by trying to minimise the *perceived* risks of medication by taking less. This is after all a logical response if you believe that the medication is necessary to control the illness yet you are simultaneously concerned about the potential adverse effects of taking it: you take some, but not all, of the recommended dose (Horne, 1997).

For many people, adherence to medication seems to be influenced by a cost–benefit analysis in which beliefs about the necessity of medication are weighed against concerns about the potential adverse effects of taking it. However, this does not imply that, each time the patient is required to take a dose of medication, s/he sits down and thinks through the pros and cons of doing so! The 'cost–benefit analysis' may be implicit rather than explicit. For example, in some situations, non-adherence could be the result of a deliberate strategy to minimise harm by taking less medication. Alternatively, it might simply be a reflection of the fact that patients who do not perceive their medication to be important may be more likely to forget to take it (Horne and Weinman, 1999).

The 'common-sense' origins of necessity beliefs and concerns

Patients' ideas about their illness and treatment are usually related to one another in a logically consistent way. This is illustrated by considering some of the correlates of necessity beliefs and concerns.

Concerns arising from suspicions of pharmaceuticals

Research has shown that many people are suspicious about medicines, perceiving them to be fundamentally harmful substances that are over-prescribed by doctors. This view is linked to wider concerns about scientific medicine, lack of trust in doctors and an increasing interest in alternative or complementary healthcare. People with a more negative orientation to medicines in general tend to have stronger concerns about the potential adverse effects of medication that has been pre-scribed for them and are consequently less adherent (Horne and Weinman, 1999).

Perceptions of specific medicines are related to more general beliefs about medicines as a whole (Horne et al., 1999). When asked to talk about medicines, people appear to access schema relating to medicines as a *class* of treatment sharing certain general properties (Echabe et al., 1992; Britten, 1994). Many patients and student volunteers have a fairly negative view of medicines as a whole, perceiving them as gener-ally harmful substances (Horne et al., 1999, 2001c). Moreover, the dangerous aspects of medication are often linked to their chemical/unnatural origins and greater concern about the potential adverse effects of prescribed medication (Horne et al., 1999) and non-adherence (Peters et al., 2001). Beliefs about medicines as a class of treatment are likely to influence a patient's expectations of a new pre-scription offered by the clinic, be they positive (e.g. 'I think it will help and is just what I need') or negative (e.g. 'I am likely to get side-effects or encounter problems with this treatment'). These initial expectations might influence how subsequent events are interpreted, for example whether symptoms are attributed to the illness or the treatment (Siegel et al., 1999). They may even influence outcome directly through the placebo/nocebo effect (see Di Blasi et al., 2003 for a review of non-specific effects).

We can only speculate on the origins of this view. One possibility is that information about a particular medicine (e.g. speculation in the press that antidepressants are 'addictive') might feed into a 'general schema' and be extrapolated to mean that 'most medicines are addictive'. Negative experiences with medicines in the past (self or significant others) are also likely to have an effect. Negative views about medicines in general appear to be related to a broader 'world-view' characterised by suspicion of chemicals in food and the environment (Gupta and Horne, 2001), and the perception that complementary therapies (e.g. homeopathy/herbalism) are more 'natural' and safer (Horne et al., 1999). This appears to be related to an increasing suspicion of science, medicine and technology within western cultures (Horne et al., 2001b; Petrie and Wessely, 2002). Suspicions of medicines, chemicals and related 'modern health worries' are associated with the use of complementary therapies and with rejection of medication (New and Senior, 1991; Gupta and Horne, 2001; Petrie et al., 2001).

Perceptions of personal sensitivity to medication

Leventhal and colleagues (personal communication, 1997) have developed a sensitive soma scale to measure individual differences in perceptions of personal sensitivity and susceptibility to the adverse effects of medication. People who view themselves as being particularly sensitive to the adverse effects of medication have stronger concerns about their prescribed medication and tend to perceive medicines in general as intrinsically harmful and overused by doctors (Horne, 1997). We know little about the origins of sensitive soma beliefs, but they may arise from more general perceptions of self and hardiness and from past experiences (of self and others).

Perceptions of personal resilience

Determining the necessity of a treatment may also be influenced by notions of self. There has been disappointingly little research in this area, but perceptions that one can resist the progress of disease by drawing on sources of 'inner strength', 'hardiness' or by keeping a 'positive outlook' emerged as reasons for rejecting HAART (highly active antiretroviral therapy) in interviews with over 100 HIV-positive men (Cooper et al., 2002). At present, we know little about the role of optimistic–pessimistic bias (the degree to which the person believes s/he is more or less at risk of a particular hazard than an 'average person') in judgements about treatment outcome and hence in treatment decisions. However, given the fairly ubiquitous effect of optimistic bias in judgements about a range of other health risks (Weinstein, 1989), it is very likely that equivalent effects will be found in relation to illness and treatments.

Perceptions of illness as origins of perceived need

Two factors appear to have a particularly strong link to patients' perceptions of the necessity of prescribed medication: their beliefs about the illness and their experience of symptoms. Patients will be more likely to agree with the necessity for prescribed medication if this accords with their perception of the illness. For example, an asthma patient who perceives his or her asthma to be a fairly short-lived problem with few personal consequences (e.g. 'I am ill when I suffer from an asthma attack but otherwise feel normal') may not have strong beliefs in the necessity of regular preventer medication and may be more inclined to manage the condition using reliever medication alone.

The effect of symptom experiences on views about medication necessity may be complex. At one level symptoms may stimulate medication use by acting as a reminder or by reinforcing beliefs about its necessity. However, patients' *expectations* of symptom relief are also likely to have an important effect. This could be problematic if the expectations are unrealistic. For example, patients who expect their newly prescribed antidepressant medication to relieve their symptoms of depression after a few doses are likely to be disappointed when they find that the medication takes several days or weeks to take any effect. This might cause them to believe that the medicine is ineffective and that continued use is not worthwhile. Symptom experience may also influence medication concerns if they are interpreted by the patient as medication side-effects.

In summary, research into patient beliefs about their illness and treatment illustrates the following key principles about the psychology of adherence.

1. Patients' beliefs about their illness and treatment are logically coherent. Although the patient's interpretation and ideas about their illness may appear mistaken from the medical perspective, they are 'common-sense' interpretations based on their own understanding and experiences.
2. Patients' behaviour (e.g. taking or not taking medication) may be more strongly influenced by their own 'common-sense' interpretation of their illness and treatment than by medical advice or instructions.
3. Patients' common-sense interpretation may be based on potentially modifiable misconceptions about the nature of the illness and about the benefits and risks of the treatment.

Information, knowledge, beliefs and behaviour

The above section has illustrated how the illness perceptions construct of Leventhal's self-regulatory model and the necessity–concerns framework might be used to operationalise patients' beliefs about illness and treatment as a basis for assessing the degree to which they match the medical view and/or the prevailing evidence. We have also discussed some of the key attributes of informed adherence. Patients' beliefs about illness and treatment are key variables but we must also consider the role of information from a range of sources (e.g. medical, internet, family, friends, media), how this is interpreted by the patient and the effect of information on knowledge and beliefs.

We have argued that patients' beliefs about medication are key to adherence decisions and have presented a simple necessity–concerns framework to show how these might be operationalised. This framework should be easy to use in practice. Clinicians could elicit patients' perceptions of their personal need for treatment and their concerns about potential adverse effects as a basis for adherence-related discussions. Beginning with a consideration of patients' perceptions of their need for the proposed treatment and their personal concerns about taking it would identify perceptual barriers to adherence. It would also help to foster a relationship in which the patient was able to contribute as a partner in the selection of treatment and the subsequent review of its effects.

However, we should not lose sight of the fact that more research is needed to complete our understanding of informed adherence. We need to know about the interactions between information, knowledge and beliefs and how these influence decision-making and adherence to prescribed medicines. Figure 7.1 shows some of the key variables that we should consider. Encouragingly, there are a number of validated methods for assessing many of these key variables (Johnston *et al.*, 1995; Bowling and Ebrahim, 2001; Cox and Mynors, 2003).

In focusing on informed adherence we should not lose sight of the importance of unintentional non-adherence. For many patients the causes of non-adherence have little to do with beliefs or preferences. They may simply forget to take their medicine or encounter practical difficulties in using it. It is important to recognise this and to develop effective ways of supporting adherence by helping patients to overcome the practical barriers to regular use of medicines (e.g. by issuing reminders, by simplifying the regimen and improving skills at using dosage devices such as inhalers).

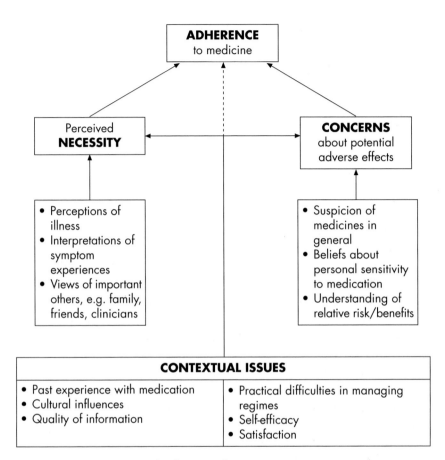

Figure 7.1   Determinants of adherence decisions

Patients as partners in treatment decisions

Recent discussions about the concordance concept have focused on the notion of partnership between patients and clinicians. In common with the concordance concept the notion of medicines partnership focuses on the clinical consultation and suggests that it should elicit patients' involvement as partners in treatment decisions (Cox and Mynors, 2003). In common with concordance, the notion of partnership needs to be more clearly defined if it is to move beyond the sound-bite to guide clinical practice (Dieppe and Horne, 2002). The process of operationalising the concept of medicines partnership has been advanced by a recent document published by the Department of Health that sets out some of the key research questions and assessment tools (Cox and Mynors, 2003).

Notions of partnership and concordance are anchored in the clinical consultation and in the effect of the consultation on patients' beliefs and behaviour. Box 7.2 lists some of the important outstanding questions relating to these issues that could be addressed in a concordance-related research agenda.

These and other concordance-related issues can be examined using the three-phase model described below.

A three-phase model for the evaluation of consultations

Concordance focuses on the consultation. Although the consultation is undoubtedly important, it is one of several influences on patients' attitudes and behaviour. Other factors should also be considered, such as how individuals process and value information from sources other than the consultation (e.g. internet, mass media, friends, family and alternative health practitioners) and how these are perceived relative to information from doctors and other healthcare professionals.

As we have already discussed, the notion of partnership is most readily understood, observed and investigated within the context of the consultation. Over the past 30 or so years, researchers have made impressive use of audio and video recording techniques to investigate

---

Box 7.2 Outstanding questions about the concept of medicines partnership

- To what extent do clinicians and patients want to work in partnership?
- What are the barriers to clinicians and patients working in partnership?
- How should we define and measure partnership? How can we recognise it when we see it?
- What are the outcomes of partnership? This should consider both subjective (e.g. satisfaction of individuals', patients' and clinicians' beliefs about the illness and treatment) and objective (e.g. effects on adherence and health outcomes) effects
- How should we identify and respond to individual differences in desires for partnership approaches to healthcare delivery?
- How can we enable patients and clinicians to work in partnership?
- What information do patients need to become active partners?

the consultation process, and to relate process variables or characteristics to outcome. Since it was difficult to make clear links between process (e.g. duration or style of consultation) and outcome variables (e.g. satisfaction, adherence, etc.), more recent studies began to examine what clinicians and patients bring to the consultation, as well as the importance of contextual factors (Stiles, 1989). Current frameworks for understanding doctor–patient communication tend to be based on the relations between *inputs* (e.g. the attitudes, beliefs, expectations and treatment preferences that patient and clinician bring to the consultation), *process* (the nature of the encounter) and *outcome* (the short- and longer-term effects on the patient) (Figure 7.2).

Input factors

Input factors which influence the consultation include not only aspects of the clinician and patient but also the context and setting in which the consultation occurs. There is now accumulating evidence that patients show consistent differences in how they want to be involved in the healthcare process (e.g. active vs. passive), and in the amount of information they would like to receive about their health problem and the proposed treatment (Horne *et al.*, 2001d).

Patients come into the healthcare setting with different levels of biomedical knowledge, based on their past experience. There is also consistent evidence that patients have differing expectations (e.g. explanation and understanding; support; medical treatment; information-seeking) for specific consultations (Williams *et al.*, 1995), and an awareness of these can be helpful in understanding not only why they are seeking help at that time but also in being able to respond effectively to their needs. Following the self-regulatory model, described earlier, it has been found that patients' illness representations will influence their decision to seek help (Cameron *et al.*, 1995) and hence their expectations of the consultation.

As outlined earlier, patients' beliefs about treatment are likely to have a profound effect on their evaluation of treatment options suggested by the clinician. An individual's attitudes towards a particular medicine will be influenced by his or her beliefs not just about that medicine but by more general views about medicines as a whole and by beliefs about potential alternatives such as complementary and alternative medicines (Furnham and Wilsmore, 1995). Here, patients' perceptions of the relative risk of treatment options (or of treatment vs. no treatment) are of fundamental importance (Bowling and Ebrahim,

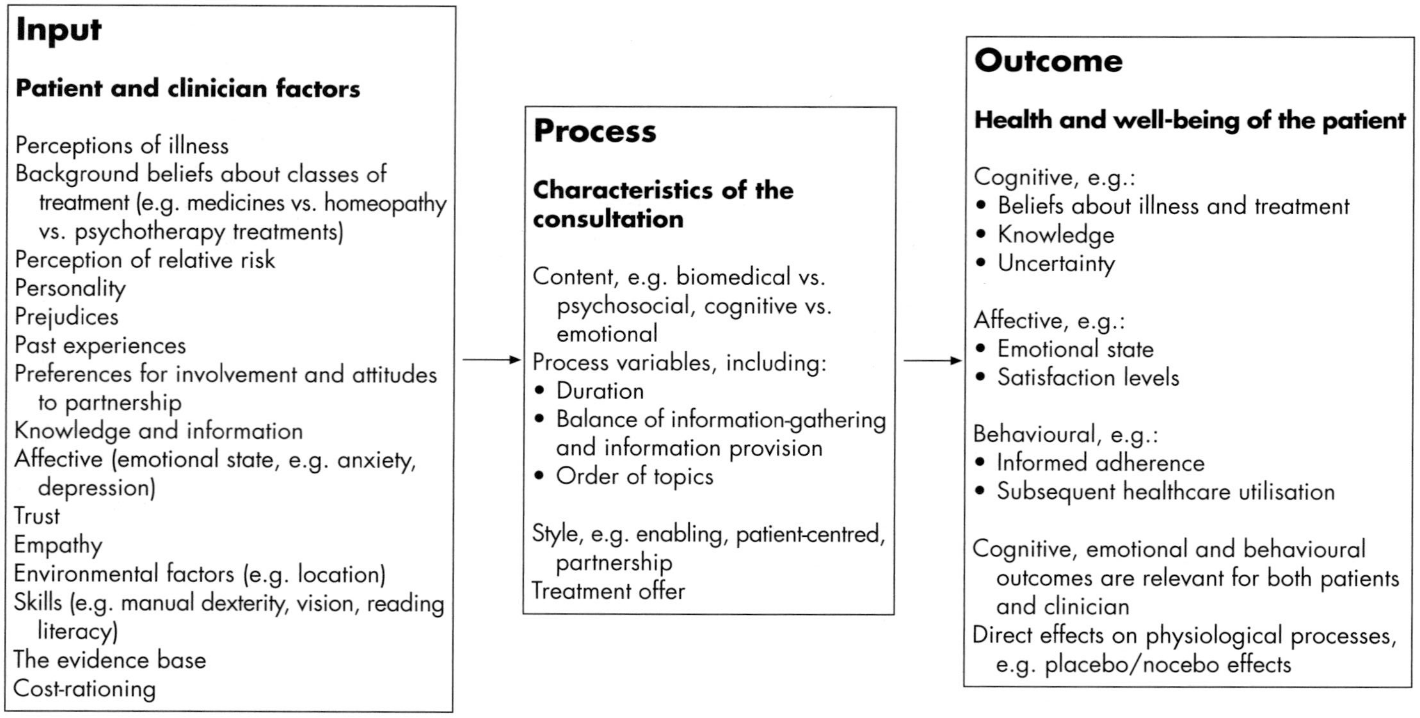

Input

Patient and clinician factors

Perceptions of illness
Background beliefs about classes of treatment (e.g. medicines vs. homeopathy vs. psychotherapy treatments)
Perception of relative risk
Personality
Prejudices
Past experiences
Preferences for involvement and attitudes to partnership
Knowledge and information
Affective (emotional state, e.g. anxiety, depression)
Trust
Empathy
Environmental factors (e.g. location)
Skills (e.g. manual dexterity, vision, reading literacy)
The evidence base
Cost-rationing

Process

Characteristics of the consultation

Content, e.g. biomedical vs. psychosocial, cognitive vs. emotional
Process variables, including:
• Duration
• Balance of information-gathering and information provision
• Order of topics

Style, e.g. enabling, patient-centred, partnership
Treatment offer

Outcome

Health and well-being of the patient

Cognitive, e.g.:
• Beliefs about illness and treatment
• Knowledge
• Uncertainty

Affective, e.g.:
• Emotional state
• Satisfaction levels

Behavioural, e.g.:
• Informed adherence
• Subsequent healthcare utilisation

Cognitive, emotional and behavioural outcomes are relevant for both patients and clinician
Direct effects on physiological processes, e.g. placebo/nocebo effects

Figure 7.2 A three-phase model for studying the effects of the consultation on medication-taking

2001). Both beliefs about treatments and perceptions of relative risk are influenced by range of personal contextual factors such as the past experiences of self and others, individuals' perceptions of what other people might want them to do, cultural norms and personality traits.

Treatment preferences will also be affected by beliefs about the self. These include beliefs about the personal sensitivity to medication as well as optimistic–pessimistic bias. Patients will also vary in their preferences for particular types of consultation and in their desires for involvement in treatment decisions (Robinson and Thomson, 2001). Also important is the degree to which the individual trusts various sources of healthcare advice such as doctors, nurses, pharmacists, government, patient support groups and the pharmaceutical industry.

Clinicians also vary considerably in the attitudes and beliefs about their own and the patient's role, and about the function and conduct of the consultation. These broad attitudinal differences are reflected in differences in the way in which the consultation is conducted (see below) and in other aspects of professional behaviour, including decision-making, prescribing and management of clinical problems. The need for clinicians to elicit and take account of their patients' preferences, beliefs and expectations is a core principle of the related concepts of concordance, patient-centredness, partnership, enablement and empowerment (see Chapter 2, this volume). Consultation begins with two sets of beliefs and values – the clinician's and the patient's. An assessment of the beliefs of patients and clinicians and the extent to which they change during or after consultation is essential to our understanding of concordance, partnership and related concepts.

The consultation process

The consultation process has been investigated using a range of methods and frameworks. A broad distinction has been made between consultations which are described as patient-centred and those which are clinician-centred (Grol *et al.*, 1990). One of the most recent consultation analysis methods is the Roter interactional analysis system (Roter *et al.*, 1997), which can identify five distinct patterns:

1. narrowly biomedical, characterised by closed-ended medical questions and biomedical talk
2. expanded biomedical, similar to the narrowly biomedical but with moderate levels of psychosocial discussion

3.   biopsychosocial, reflecting a balance of psychosocial and biomedical topics
4.   psychosocial, characterised by psychosocial exchange
5.   consumerist, characterised by patient questions and doctor information–giving

Another approach to process analysis can be found in the studies of Phillip Ley (1988), who concentrated on the informational content of the consultation and the quality of information provided by the doctor. In particular they have analysed the content in terms of its level of complexity, comprehensibility and the extent to which the information is organised. They have found that if medical information is too detailed or complex, important information may not be understood, retained or acted upon by the patient.

These various ways of conceptualising and analysing the consultation process have given rise to a large number of indices or categories that have been related to outcomes, often in quite a limited fashion. Outcomes such as patient satisfaction or adherence to treatment are likely to be determined by a range of factors, reflecting a complex interaction of input, process and situational variables.

Outcomes of healthcare communication

For healthcare communication, important outcomes include health, well-being and satisfaction but only relatively few studies have measured short- or longer-term health outcomes following consultations. From the patient's perspective consultation outcomes fall into three broad groups: (1) *cognitive* (changes in knowledge, understanding and beliefs); (2) *affective* (emotional state, satisfaction levels); and (3) *behavioural* (changes in health-related behaviour, including adherence to treatment or advice). The cognitive, affective and behavioural outcomes of the consultation are very closely linked and can influence each other. Patient satisfaction, understanding and beliefs can play a major role in influencing adherence with treatment or advice, which is obviously important in situations where non-adherence results in adverse health consequences. Since there is evidence of high levels of non-adherence, this can clearly affect other outcomes including health and well-being. The consultation and relationship between clinician and patient may also have a direct effect on health outcomes by contributing to the non-specific effects of treatment underlying the placebo and nocebo effects (Di Blasi *et al.*, 2003).

Conceptualising medication-related consultations as a three-phase process has implications for the assessment and evaluation of concordance. The need to take account of input, process and output variables suggests that assessment will require a combination of approaches and tools. The need for a better understanding of the consultation, as well as the need to assess the impact of different processes on outcomes, will demand a combination of qualitative and quantitative approaches. It is unlikely that a single assessment tool or questionnaire will be sufficient to evaluate the concept of concordance. Rather, assessment could proceed by defining key input, process and output indicators and selecting tools to measure these. In some cases new approaches may need to be developed and validated. However, many of the key variables may be assessed using existing, validated methods (Johnston *et al.*, 1995; Bowling *et al.*, 2001; Cox and Mynors, 2003).

Summary and conclusions

Good prescribing is about more than pharmacology. It is represents a compromise between two value systems: the scientific evidence base which determines the most safe and (cost-) effective option for treatment and the patient's common-sense beliefs about the illness and treatment. The difficulty comes when there is conflict between these and intentional non-adherence is the result. Concordance appears to deal with this by suggesting that the patient's view predominates. However, many 'patient-centred' clinicians will be uncomfortable with this solution if they perceive the patients' views to be based on mistaken beliefs or misconceptions about the illness and treatment.

A pragmatic alternative, which is consistent with the spirit of concordance, is to use 'informed adherence' as the guiding principle. Here the role of the practitioner is to help ensure that the patient's decision about using medicines can be informed by a realistic assessment of the likely benefits and risks rather than by potentially misplaced beliefs or myths. To do this, practitioners will need to elicit patients' views but also to challenge and try to change beliefs that they consider to be based on misconceptions or erroneous interpretations of the evidence. To assist patients to self-manage chronic illness by getting the best from medicines, clinicians could adopt a perceptions and practicalities approach (Horne, 2001) to facilitate informed adherence. To do this they will need to elicit and help reduce both the perceptual barriers (e.g. potentially misplaced beliefs about the illness and about the relative risks and benefits of treatment options) and the practical barriers (e.g.

poor comprehension, forgetting, regimen complexity) to informed adherence to evidence-based prescriptions.

We are still left with the problem of uncertainty in medicine. Most prescribing decisions are, to some extent, therapeutic experiments. Treatment choices are guided by assumptions about likely risks and benefit based on an extrapolation of the results of group effects from clinical trials to the unique situation of the individual. The challenge for clinicians is to present the medical rationale for prescription in a way which can be understood by the patient and to identify and attempt to correct misconceptions that might act as a barrier to achieving an improved quality of life. Having done this, the patient's 'informed decision' should be respected but cannot necessarily be supported (e.g. if it conflicts with the greater good).

The concept of concordance has placed a consideration of patients' beliefs and preferences at the centre of the debate on how to improve healthcare. Finding better ways of helping patients and clinicians to work in partnership to achieve informed adherence to evidence-based prescriptions is a priority for medicines-related research. This chapter has outlined a philosophical and practical approach to the development of a research agenda to achieve this.

References

Arluke A (1980). Judging drugs: patients' conceptions of therapeutic efficacy in the treatment of arthritis. *Hum Org* 39: 84–88.

Bowling A, Ebrahim S (2001). Measuring patients' preferences for treatment and perceptions of risk. *Qual Health Care* 10: i2–i8.

Britten N (1994). Patients' ideas about medicines: a qualitative study in a general practice population. *Br J Gen Pract* 44: 465–468.

Cameron L, Leventhal E A, Leventhal H (1995). Seeking medical care in response to symptoms and life stress. *Psychosom Med* 57: 37–47.

Campbell M, Fitzpatrick R, Haines A *et al.* (2000). Framework for design and evaluation of complex interventions to improve health. *BMJ* 321: 694–696.

Conner M, Norman P (1996). *Predicting Health Behaviour*. Buckingham: Open University Press.

Cooper V, Horne R, Gellaitry G *et al.* (2002). Perceptions of HAART among HIV-positive men who have been recommended treatment. *HIV Med* 3: 157–194.

Coulter A (1985). Decision-making and the pill: the consumer's view. *Br J Fam Planning* 11: 98–103.

Cox K, Mynors G (2003). *Project Evaluation Toolkit*. London: Medicines Partnership.

Di Blasi Z, Harkness E, Ernst E *et al.* (2003). Influence of context effects on health outcomes: a systematic review. *Lancet* 357: 757–762.

Dieppe P, Horne R (2002). Soundbites and patient centred care. *BMJ* 325: 605.

Echabe A E, Guillen C S, Ozmaiz J A (1992). Representations of health, illness and medicines: coping strategies and health promoting behaviour. *Br J Clin Psychol* 31: 339–349.

Furnham V C, Wilsmore M (1995). The perceived efficacy of complementary and orthodox medicine among complementary and general practice patients. *Health Educ Res* 10: 395–405.

Gabe J, Lipshitz Phillips S (1982). Evil necessity? The meaning of benzodiazepine use for women patients from one general practice. *Sociol Health Illness* 4: 201–209.

Gill A, Williams A C (2001). Preliminary study of chronic pain patients' concerns about cannabinoids as analgesics. *Clin J Pain* 17: 245–248.

Grol R, de Maeseneer J, Whitfield M, Mokkink H (1990). Disease-centred versus patient-centred attitudes: a comparison of general practitioners in Belgium, Britain and the Netherlands. *Fam Pract* 7: 100–104.

Gupta K, Horne R (2001). The influence of health beliefs on the presentation and consultation outcome in patients with chemical sensitivities. *J Psychosom Res* 50: 131–137.

Hand C H, Bradley C (1996). Health beliefs of adults with asthma: toward an understanding of the difference between symptomatic and preventive use of inhaler treatment. *J Asthma* 33: 331–338.

Haynes R B, McKibbon K A, Kanani R (1996). Systematic review of randomised clinical trials of interventions to assist patients to follow prescriptions for medications. *Lancet* 348: 383–386.

Horne R (1997). Representations of medication and treatment: advances in theory and measurement. In: Petrie K J, Weinman J A (eds) *Perceptions of Health and Illness: Current Research and Applications*. London: Harwood Academic Press, 155–188.

Horne R (1998). Adherence to medication: a review of existing research. In: Myers L, Midence K (eds) *Adherence to Treatment in Medical Conditions*. London: Harwood Academic, 285–310.

Horne R (2001). Compliance, adherence and concordance. In: Taylor K, Harding G (eds) *Pharmacy Practice*. London: Taylor and Francis, 165–184.

Horne R (2003). Treatment perceptions and self regulation. In: Cameron L D, Leventhal H (eds) *The Self-Regulation of Health and Illness Behaviour*. London: Routledge, 138–153.

Horne R, Weinman J (1998). Predicting treatment adherence: an overview of theoretical models. In: Myers L, Midence K (eds) *Adherence to Treatment in Medical Conditions*. London: Harwood Academic, 25–50.

Horne R, Weinman J (1999). Patients' beliefs about prescribed medicines and their role in adherence to treatment in chronic physical illness. *J Psychosom Res* 47: 555–567.

Horne R, Weinman J (2002). Self regulation and self management in asthma: exploring the role of illness perceptions and treatment beliefs in explaining non-adherence to preventer medication. *Psychol Health* 00 (1): 21.

Horne R, Weinman J, Hankins M (1999). The Beliefs about Medicines Questionnaire: the development and evaluation of a new method for assessing the cognitive representation of medication. *Psychol Health* 14: 1–24.

Horne R, Sumner S, Jubraj B *et al.* (2001a). Haemodialysis patients' beliefs about treatment: implications for adherence to medication and dietary/fluid restrictions. *Int J Pharm Pract* 9: 169–175.

Horne R, Cooper V, Fisher M, Buick D (2001b). Beliefs about HIV and HAART and the decision to accept or reject HAART. Seventh Annual Meeting of the British HIV Association (BHIVA), 27–29 April 2001, Brighton, UK. *HIV Med* 2: 195.

Horne R, Frost S, Hankins M, Wright S (2001c). "In the eye of the beholder": pharmacy students have more positive perceptions of medicines than students of other disciplines. *Int J Pharm Pract* 9: 85–89.

Horne R, Hankins M, Jenkins R (2001d). The Satisfaction with Information about Medicines Scale (SIMS): a new measurement tool for audit and research. *Qual Health Care* 10: 135–140.

Horne R, Cooper V, Gellaitry G *et al.* (2002). Predicting acceptance of highly active antiretroviral treatment (HAART): the role of patients' perceptions of illness and treatment. In: *Proceedings of the XIV International AIDS Conference*. Barcelona, Spain, July 7–12.

Horne R, Buick D, Fisher M *et al.* (2004). Doubts about necessity and concerns about adverse effects: identifying the types of beliefs that are associated with non-adherence to HAART. *Int J STD AIDS* 15: 38–44.

Horton R (2003). The dis-eases of medicine. In: *Second Opinion: Doctors, Diseases and Decisions in Modern Medicine*. London: Granta Publications, 1–61.

Johnston M, Wright S, Weinman J (1995). *Measures in Health Psychology: A User's Portfolio*. Oxford: NFER-Nelson.

Leventhal H, Diefenbach M, Leventhal E A (1992). Illness cognition: using common sense to understand treatment adherence and affect cognition interactions. Special issue: cognitive perspectives in health psychology. *Cogn Ther Res* 16: 143–163.

Ley P (1988). *Communicating with Patients*. London: Chapman & Hall.

McGavock H (1996). *A Review of the Literature on Drug Adherence*. London: Royal Pharmaceutical Society of Great Britain/Merck Sharp & Dohme.

Michie S, Dormandy E, Marteau T M (2003). Informed choice: understanding knowledge in the context of screening uptake. *Patient Educ Couns* 50: 247–253.

Morgan M, Watkins C J (1988). Managing hypertension: beliefs and responses to medication among cultural groups. *Sociol Health Illness* 10: 561–578.

New S J, Senior M L (1991). 'I don't believe in needles': qualitative aspects of a study into the uptake of immunisation in two English health authorities. *Soc Sci Med* 33: 509–518.

Peters K F, Horne R, Kong F *et al.* (2001). Living with Marfan syndrome 2. Medication adherence and physical activity modification. *Clin Genet* 60: 283–292.

Petrie K J, Wessely S (2002). Modern worries, new technology, and medicine. *BMJ* 324: 690–691.

Petrie K J, Sivertsen B, Hysing M *et al.* (2001). Thoroughly modern worries: the relationship of worries about modernity to reported symptoms, health and medical care utilization. *J Psychosom Res* 51: 395–401.

Robinson A, Thomson R (2001). Variability in patient preferences for participating in medical decision making: implication for the use of decision support tools. *Qual Health Care* 10: i34–i38.

Roter D L, Stewart M, Putnam S M, Lipkin M Jr (1997). Communication patterns of primary care physicians. *JAMA* 277: 350–356.

Royal Pharmaceutical Society of Great Britain (1997). *From Compliance to Concordance: Achieving Shared Goals in Medicine Taking*. London: RPSGB.

Siegel K, Dean L, Schrimshaw E W (1999). Symptom ambiguity among late-middle-aged and older adults with HIV. *Res Ageing* 21: 595–618.

Stiles W B (1989). Evaluating medical interview process components: null correlations with outcomes may be misleading. *Med Care* 27 (2): 212–220.

Webb D G, Horne R, Pinching A J (2001). Treatment-related empowerment: preliminary evaluation of a new measure in patients with advanced HIV disease. *Int J STD AIDS* 12: 103–107.

Weinstein N D (1989). Effects of personal experience on self-protective behavior. *Psychol Bull* 105: 31–50.

Williams S, Weinman J, Dale J, Newman S (1995). Patient expectations; what do primary care patients want from the GP and how far does meeting expectations affect patient satisfaction? *Fam Pract* 12: 193–201.

World Health Organization (2003). *Adherence to Long-Term Therapies: Evidence for Action*. Geneva: World Health Organization.

8

A policy framework for concordance

Joanne Shaw

Introduction

In April 2001 the Health Minister, Lord Hunt, signalled a new chapter in the concordance project by committing £1.3m over 2 years to a Joint Task Force to work towards implementing the concept of concordance within the NHS. The Task Force came together for the first time in January 2002 and, at the time of writing, is precisely half-way through its 2-year programme. This first year of the Task Force on Medicines Partnership – as it was named – offers perhaps the best indication of how concordance is likely to develop over the coming years and an idea of what some of the most significant future challenges are likely to be.

It is worth noting that the Task Force began its work without a clear, evidence-based picture of what concordance might look like in practice or the benefits it might produce for patients and the NHS. These have been discussed in more detail in earlier chapters. Concordance is without doubt a very powerful concept. The continued scale and ubiquity of non-compliance with prescribed medication, and the combined failure of health professionals, the NHS and the pharmaceutical industry to solve the problem, are in themselves highly persuasive arguments in favour of concordance (Medicines Partnership, 2003). There are many individual studies attesting to the significance of patient–health professional communication and the importance of patients' attitudes and beliefs about medicine as an influence on their medicine-taking behaviour. Sadly, this does not add up to a watertight proof of concordance, still less a blueprint for how to implement it.

It was a brave step to jump from theory straight to implementation, so at the start of this new phase the key questions were: what could realistically be achieved in 2 years and, given the inevitable constraints, how should the time best be used to position concordance for the future?

Definitions

In one sense, the inheritance of the new Task Force on Medicines Partnership consisted, in addition to the budget, of some people, a concept and a definition. But anything beyond a cursory consideration of the definition, interesting and radical as it was, revealed problems. For example, was concordance meant to be a process or an outcome? According to the strict definition given in the original report, known by many as the Green Book (Royal Pharmaceutical Society of Great Britain, 1997), it was an outcome, but proponents clearly used the term to mean process (in the construction 'concordant consultation', for example). And while the definition spoke of 'an alliance in which the health care professionals recognise the primacy of the patient's decisions', it was not meant as a serious proposal that patients should be prescribed any medicine they asked for (albeit anecdotal evidence suggests that many hard-pressed GPs do exactly that). Medicines Partnership took the definition as a starting point. Other things were also needed to support the transition from theory into practice. A tripartite framework was developed to encapsulate the elements needed to 'operationalise' concordance. The model depicts three constituent elements that are needed to put concordance into practice:

1.   patients having access to the information, knowledge and skills they need to participate as partners in prescribing decisions
2.   prescribing consultations involving patients as partners in shared decisions about treatment
3.   patients supported in taking their medicines according to the concordant agreement that has been made

These are illustrated in Figure 8.1.

No model is perfect. But this one has proved surprisingly useful and durable, both as a communication tool, with lay people and health professionals, and as a guide to implementing concordance, with practitioners and managers.

The political context

In bridging the theoretical and the practical, the 'three-pillars' model reminds us of how far the world has moved on since the notion of concordance first emerged as the answer to questions, specifically about *medicines*. The purpose of the initial inquiry that led to the publication of the Green Book was to investigate why so much medicine is not taken

CONCORDANCE
a process of prescribing and
medicine-taking based on partnership

Patients have enough knowledge to participate as partners	Prescribing consultations involve patients as partners	Patients are supported in taking medicines
• Patients are offered information about medicines which is clear, accurate, accessible and sufficiently detailed • The information provided is tailored to individual patients' needs • Education programmes empower patients to take responsibility for their own health	• Patients are invited to talk about their priorities, preferences and concerns about medicine-taking and the proposed treatment, and these are explored openly • Professionals explain the rationale for, and the characteristics of, the proposed treatment • Patients and health professionals jointly agree on a course of treatment which reconciles as far as possible the professional's recommendations and the patient's preferences • The patient's and professional's understanding of what has been agreed is checked • The patient's ability to follow the agreed treatment is checked	• All appropriate opportunities are used to discuss medicines issues (e.g. patients' interactions with doctors, pharmacists and nurses) • Health professionals share medicines information effectively with each other • Medications are reviewed regularly, with patients' participation • Practical difficulties in taking medicines are addressed

Figure 8.1   The three pillars of concordance

as prescribed, and what can be done about it. Since then, however, the broader health policy agenda has in one sense 'caught up' with concordance, which can now claim deeper resonance beyond the realm of medicines. It sits, in fact, at a particularly interesting confluence between the medicines agenda from whence it came, and two other dominant policy streams: patient and public involvement on the one hand and the patient safety agenda on the other. If concordance is to capture the professional and public imagination it will have to advance beyond the relatively narrow confines of what might be called the pure medicines agenda. For that to happen we need to understand how concordance can help take forward both of these other agendas; identify and capitalise on overlaps; and look for ways to achieve shared goals.

If one reads carefully between the lines, the way the new Task Force on Medicines Partnership was constituted and positioned revealed both how concordance was, and perhaps still is, viewed in the Department of Health, and the political context into which it was born.

Firstly, Medicines Partnership was positioned squarely in the realm of medicines, pharmacy and industry, under the umbrella of *Pharmacy in the Future* (Department of Health, 2001a). This sets it alongside very different initiatives such as electronic transfer of prescriptions, repeat dispensing and the National Prescribing Centre's national collaborative Medicines Management Services programme, all of which are more about improving the mechanics of medicines management processes and systems than about cultural change. At the same time, this left concordance without a very clear link to the developing patient and public involvement arena to which, conceptually, it is strongly aligned.

Secondly, the Task Force as a body was established as a very broad church. Clearly it needed to represent the health professions, the Department and the NHS. But it also brought together the pharmaceutical industry, the academics and, crucially, patient groups, as equal members. This breadth of representation is relatively unusual and creates its own challenges. On the one hand it provides a uniquely powerful platform for innovation by bringing together a range of perspectives to inform and challenge one another. On the other, it may make progress more difficult to achieve. This is due partly to inherent differences in perspectives which might obstruct consensus and partly due to the resultant expectations of progress across a very broad front which have the potential to dilute focus and energy, and limit overall achievement. On balance, however, this breadth has proved to be a huge advantage compared with many professionally driven NHS programmes, where clinical and managerial agendas typically dominate, industry voice is rarely heard, and patient involvement is heavily outweighed by professional perspectives.

The third interesting aspect of the Task Force's remit and initial programme is the implicit approach to change management that it embodied. The government's overall thinking on change management can best be described as evolving. Point to any handful of public service improvement initiatives and you are likely to find a different underlying change management logic for each one. Some represent strong, centrally driven reform, with a single template, rigorously applied around the country with little or no scope for local tailoring or ownership by the front-line staff responsible for implementation. The national literacy strategy (Department for Education and Skills, 2003) and the Expert Patient programme (Department of Health, 2001b) are both examples of this method. Others follow an equally strong but entirely different 'bottom-up' methodology, in which central direction is restricted to setting the measures to be collected, and improvement relies exclusively on small-cycle change based on local innovation, supported by a combination of best practice sharing and competitive spirit. The national collaborative Medicines Management Services programme is one example, and there are several other well-established collaborative programmes addressing various aspects of NHS performance, including cancer and access to primary care. Still other improvement initiatives use a judicious mixture of central guidance and local experimentation to achieve step changes in performance, such as a current programme to restructure the school workforce.

There is no single blueprint for successful change management. It is likely that different approaches work best in different circumstances depending on factors such as certainty about the solution, the extent of improvement required and the speed of change in the external environment (Audit Commission, 2001). The important thing is to consider the strengths and weaknesses of alternative approaches explicitly, and match the methodology selected to the requirements of the situation. Unfortunately, this seldom appears to happen.

The change management approach implicit in the initial Task Force programme, to the extent that one is discernible, can perhaps best be described as professional development-based, in that it appears to envisage educating health professionals in concordance as the primary engine for change. Thus, professional development is the largest single line item in the initial budget and the only one with dedicated staff resources attached. One obvious implication of this approach is its impact on the timescale in which results can be expected. Change that relies on education is inevitably a long-term enterprise whose results are more likely to be observed over many years rather than a period of 24 months.

A final environmental factor that fundamentally affects the potential for implementing concordance in practice is the powerful sense within the NHS of being overwhelmed by programmes, targets, impera-tives and 'must do's' – sometimes referred to as initiative overload. Even the recent generous resource allocation for the NHS has increased the perceived pressure to deliver improvements within very real capacity constraints. In an environment where failing to meet waiting-time targets can and does bring management careers to an end, putting yet another item on the local delivery agenda is an enormous challenge.

The Task Force programme

The Task Force programme highlights five themes. Individual Task Force activities, such as the guide to medication review (Medicines Partnership, 2002), cut across these themes and contribute in different ways to their achievement.

- *Professional development*: influencing the education and professional development of doctors, nurses and pharmacists to equip them with the attitudes, knowledge and skills to implement concordance in their profes-sional practice
- *Communication*: communicating with and supporting patients and the public with medicine-taking and helping them to develop a better under-standing and awareness of their medicines
- *Policy:* working with policy-makers and related groups such as the National Institute for Clinical Excellence (NICE) to ensure that patient partnership and concordance are embedded in the design and delivery of key policy initiatives
- *Research and development:* drawing on the existing evidence base to identify strategies for putting concordance into practice and developing approaches to measure and audit results
- *Pilots and model practice*: demonstrating the potential for putting con-cordance into practice and producing measurable benefits within the NHS

The remainder of this chapter is spent reviewing progress in each of these areas and considering the implications for the future of concord-ance.

Progress to date and future developments

Professional development

The goal of building concordance into the education, training and pro-fessional development of doctors, nurses and pharmacists has proven to be a major challenge, particularly in medicine (White, 2003). The professional development remit could be interpreted very broadly to include potentially undergraduate, pre- and postregistration training, as well as continuing professional development. With very limited resources at its disposal, the Task Force undertook a structured mapping exercise to analyse the different education and training systems operating within each profession and identify where the Task Force could have the greatest impact. This led to a focus on the postgraduate levels. The Task Force was committed from its inception to delivering 90 'concordance leaders' or 'champions' across the three prescribing professions, following a model previously used successfully in GP education. Interest in these roles – now called concordance facilitators – has not been uniform across the professions. Of the current group of 60 professional (as opposed to lay) facilitators, 30 are pharmacists, 20 nurses and 10 doctors. Experience to date has indicated that, while pharmacists as a group already appeared to have a relatively well-developed awareness (a search of the *Pharmaceutical Journal* archive brings up 144 references to concordance before 1 January 2002), if not understanding, of concordance, this was not replicated across the other two groups.

The degree to which concordance has been adopted within existing curricula also varies between the professions and across different academic institutions. Concordance is very much in evidence in the extended prescribing training for nurses. But while, for example, in Aberdeen, concordance features heavily in the undergraduate medicine communications skills course, in London it is possible to train and qualify as a doctor without ever having heard the word 'concordance'. Over the remaining life of the Task Force, it will be critically important to develop a better understanding of the pressures and development agendas within each profession, if concordance is to be successfully grafted on to existing structures and processes beyond 2003, without the benefit of a centrally supported team.

The process being followed by the Task Force to deliver its professional development objectives involves recruiting the required number of concordance facilitators from each profession, targeting individuals who have professional development or educational roles, and preparing them to teach concordance. Preparation takes the form of a 1-day workshop developed and taught, mostly in small multidisciplinary groups, by leading figures in GP, nurse and pharmacy education. Delegates to this workshop will go on to experiment with teaching concordance themselves, and come together again after a period of a few months to share their experiences as the basis for preparing the next phase.

Given the nature of the concordance concept, it is imperative that the patient perspective runs through every aspect of the implementation phase, including what is known as 'professional' development. The professional development programme therefore involves patients at every stage. There are patient representatives within the core tutor group designing and teaching the first workshop for concordance facilitators. The recruitment process targeted patient representatives to become concordance facilitators and participate on equal terms at the preparatory workshop. This is possible because most of those patient representatives are expected to be lay tutors from patient self-management courses, i.e. teachers themselves, in the same way as their professional counterparts.

It will be fascinating to see how the Task Force professional development programme evolves over the next few months. The way that it is currently structured combines some teaching methods that have been tried and tested with health professionals over many years, together with other genuinely new elements. Although patients have been involved in medical education and assessment for many years, this particular model of equal involvement of patient representatives as teachers and learners alongside health professionals from several disciplines is unusual.

It is too early so say whether this approach will be fully successful, if success is measured in terms of the long-term integration of concordance within mainstream teaching for the doctors, nurses and pharmacists of the future. The barriers to success are daunting, and are underlined by the difficulties the Task Force has experienced in recruiting the very modest numbers of concordance facilitators required for this phase of the programme. However, it seems certain that the programme will provide a significantly new and better understanding of how health professionals and patients can be brought together as equal partners in training, education and development within the NHS. This is an example of where the influence of the Task Force on Medicines Partnership is likely to stretch well beyond its principal focus of implementing the concordance concept, through an important and broader contribution towards a more patient-centred health service.

Communication

Assuring a successful future for concordance requires building awareness and communicating key messages about concordance to target audiences of health professionals, the NHS, the pharmaceutical industry, politicians and patient groups. A number of articles about concordance in practice, the work of the Task Force and specific publications such as the guide to medication review have been published in professional journals since January 2002 (Marinker and Shaw, 2003). In parallel, an active programme of outreach and networking has been pursued with stakeholder groups and opinion leaders in the NHS and beyond.

There is, however, a bigger communication agenda for concordance, beyond the essential ongoing dialogue with stakeholders and decision-makers. To establish genuine partnership between patients and health professionals in relation to medicines requires a major, sustained effort at communicating with the public, to prepare the 'patient side' of the concordance partnership. The public needs to be invited and supported to find out more about their own medicines and encouraged to express their beliefs, attitudes and preferences about medicines to health professionals.

This is only achievable through a major public awareness campaign, involving a broad range of stakeholders and probably repeated and refined over a number of years. By the time this book is published, the first Ask About Medicines Week will have taken place, under the leadership of an executive group including the Task Force on Medicines Partnership. Although to some extent modelled on similar campaigns in the USA, Australia and Scandinavia, the crucial difference between these and the UK initiative is the UK's core focus on concordance, with patient safety a key but subsidiary benefit.

Ask About Medicines Week is potentially a route towards delivering concordance in practice on a wide scale, in an accelerated timescale. Thus it complements the Task Force professional development programme which, in the first instance, focuses on equipping a relatively small and select group with concordance skills. The success of Ask About Medicines Week depends upon stimulating public demand for information and dialogue about medicines, and at the same time providing effective channels for meeting the demand, with informed, willing and available health professionals and a range of accessible, objective, patient-friendly sources of information about medicines.

It is not only Ask About Medicines Week that depends for its success on improving medicines information for the public; the entire concordance enterprise requires it. Good medicines information is a key building block for concordance. It is impossible to imagine genuine partnership between health professionals and patients in relation to medicines decisions as long as access to high-quality information about medicines is only available to patients through the medium of a health professional.

Medicines information for the public is a highly contentious arena. The form and content of publicly available information about prescription medicines are tightly regulated at a European level. Attempts to liberalise medicines information are hampered by fears of a slippery slope towards unfettered direct-to-consumer advertising. At the same time, the one area of unanimous agreement is the unsatisfactory state of the current statutory patient information leaflet. As Raynor has noted, patient information leaflets are too narrow, too negative and too late to be really useful to patients (Anonymous, 2003). The upshot is thus the paradoxical situation in which technologically literate consumers can find unregulated medicines information from anywhere on the globe through the medium of the internet, while the rest are reliant on a patient information leaflet which is widely perceived to be unhelpful and inadequate (Raynor *et al.*, 2003).

Breaking this deadlock would be a significant step towards putting in place one of the key building blocks required for concordance. The goal would be to provide clear, objective, evidence-based information about prescription medicines for people who actively seek it out. It would require radically new thinking, the starting point being what patients and the public want and have a right to know, as opposed to what pharmaceutical companies would like to be able to tell them, or what governments would or would not like them to have access to. With its patient, NHS, Department of Health and industry representation, the Task Force on Medicines Partnership is ideally positioned to take the lead in this area and to help facilitate a practical solution with which all parties can feel comfortable. This is most likely to happen as a result of the impetus provided by Ask About Medicines Week. It could be one of the most valuable achievements of the Task Force and a powerful contribution to the realisation of concordance.

Policy

Active work with policy-makers during 2002 has confirmed that, on the whole, concordance has yet to make an impact on other aspects of health policy. In other words, individual policy strands have not yet recognised medicine-taking as a significant issue nor, therefore, begun to consider how to achieve partnership in prescribing decisions for specific conditions or patient groups. The role of the Task Force on Medicines Partnership has therefore been to work with the Department of Health and other organisations to raise awareness of medicine-taking issues and to ensure that concordance is embedded within the development and delivery of key policy initiatives.

During the first year of the Task Force, contact was made with most policy development initiatives where concordance is relevant. These include the National Service Frameworks (NSFs), NICE and the extension of prescribing responsibilities (Department of Health, 2003). The logic for considering concordance within NSFs and NICE guidelines is that expected benefits for implementing new treatment standards and guidelines are unlikely to materialise unless compliance issues are tackled within core standards and guidance. It is vital for policy-makers to realise that, unless there is real agreement between the patient and the health professional about the treatment to be followed, a significant proportion of medicines, perhaps half, perhaps more, will not be taken as prescribed (Royal Pharmaceutical Society of Great Britain, 1997). This will inevitably undermine any investment that is made as a result of new policies, in setting treatment standards and developing better health services. The challenge for the Task Force is to provide sufficient evidence of the impact of concordance to carry conviction amongst clinical experts in an environment where policy-making is becoming ever more rigorously evidence-based.

The importance of concordance in relation to the extension of prescribing responsibilities is the opportunity that now exists to influence a new generation of nurse and pharmacist prescribers so that concordance becomes integral to their practice from the very outset of their prescribing careers. The mechanism for introducing concordance to this group potentially exists in the mandatory training that new prescribers from both professions will be required to undertake before they are allowed to prescribe. This is being picked up through the Task Force's professional development programme, described above, by targeting people involved in nurse and pharmacist prescribing training as concordance facilitators.

In its first few months, the Task Force was involved in a Management of Medicines Group attached to the Renal NSF. The group was responsible for identifying the key medicines issues for renal treatment and submitted a paper to the NSF External Reference Group in summer 2002. The experience of working with this group highlighted a number of interesting issues for embedding concordance within other health policies:

• Each policy development team of civil servants and external experts has its own particular character and concerns, driven partly by the specific backgrounds and interests of the individuals who happen to be involved. Policy-making can therefore be a more personalised and less purely objective process than it might appear from the outside.

- The views of different policy development groups on medicines and how they are best used are not consistent.
- Some policy development groups regard medicines issues as a relatively minor, insignificant aspect of medical care and are far more concerned, for example, with service configuration – who should do what, where.
- Even those who believe that medicines are important, including specialist pharmacists, for example, tend to adopt a strongly technical perspective which does not naturally encompass consideration of patients' views on medicines and medicine-taking. This may reflect the fact that such policy groups tend to be dominated by experts from specialist departments in hospitals, where medicines are administered under supervision and non-compliance is therefore less of a problem than in primary care.

As a result of the work of the Renal NSF medicines group, a need was identified for a 'generic' Management of Medicines Group to support a number of NSFs in development. This should improve the consistency with which medicines issues are considered by the various NSF teams and reduce the amount of duplication involved in separate groups supporting each individual NSF. However, it is reasonable to assume that convincing the various External Reference Groups who are developing NSFs of the importance of medicine-taking and concordance will remain a considerable task for the foreseeable future.

The best example so far of an NSF that has given serious consideration to medicines is the NSF for Older People (OPNSF), which was published with a supplement dedicated to medicines management issues (Department of Health, 2001c). Given that four out of five people over 75 years of age take prescription medicines and 36% take four or more, this was a very important document. It recommended that everyone over 75 should have their medicines reviewed annually, or twice a year for people taking four or more different medicines. This became an explicit milestone for the implementation of the NSF, to be achieved by every primary care trust (PCT) by April 2002.

The OPNSF medicines management booklet did not, however, provide a definition of what qualifies as a medication review, nor guidance about how reviews were to be implemented or recorded. Consequently there was a great deal of activity in general practices and PCTs around the country aimed at meeting the NSF milestone, but widely different interpretations of what medication reviews should consist of and how they should be provided. Nor were there consistent data which the Department of Health could use to judge progress and determine whether the milestone had been achieved.

Medication review provided an important opportunity for the Task Force to promote the practical application of concordance outside its core group of enthusiasts by providing much-needed practical guidance for practitioners about how to implement medication reviews. This could potentially have been done equally successfully by quite a number of well-qualified bodies, including the Department of Health itself. The importance of the initiative being led by the Task Force on Medicines Partnership was that it enabled the implementation of medication reviews to become a vehicle for applying concordance in practice. This was achieved by basing the definition and principles of medication review used in the guide on the concept of concordance, and by researching the needs of older people, patients and carers to inform the guidance (Medicines Partnership, 2002). This resulted in a guide that was palpably different from the kind of technocratic 'safety–efficacy–cost-effectiveness' document that would have been the more likely product had it been developed by other possible authors.

This example highlights the importance of identifying and seizing opportunities to advance concordance as they present themselves. It also underlines the importance of working in partnership with complementary organisations and programmes. The medication review guide was produced jointly by the Task Force and the national collaborative Medicines Management Services programme. The partnership resulted in a powerful combination of principle and pragmatism, as well as providing essential credibility with practitioners that comes from the practical grounding of the Medicines Management Services programme.

The widespread implementation of medication review according to a concordance model will hopefully act as a showcase for concordance in practice. The implementation of concordant medication reviews may be used by the Commission for Health Improvement (soon to become the Commission for Health Audit and Inspection, CHAI) in its approach to clinical governance reviews of PCTs. It is a useful marker of a number of aspects of PCT performance in which CHAI is interested, including quality of care, use of resources and patient involvement. The hope is that it will also demonstrate how concordance can be successfully integrated into policy implementation, thereby opening the door for consideration of concordance in other aspects of health policy.

In addition to policies about specific conditions and patient groups, such as the NSFs and the Chief Medical Officer's Epilepsy Action Plan (Department of Health, personal communication) the two high-profile policy streams with which concordance has the closest affinity are patient safety and patient and public involvement.

Patient safety became a high-profile issue in the UK with the publication of *An Organisation with a Memory* (Department of Health, 2001d). That led directly to the establishment of the National Patient Safety Agency with its remit to set up comprehensive incident-reporting systems throughout the NHS to enable the service to monitor and learn from mistakes and near-misses. Medication errors make up a significant proportion of untoward incidents within the health service, though in the absence of a comprehensive and reliable database it is difficult to say precisely what the real number of medicines errors might be. Mistakes may happen at any stage of the process: prescribing, dispensing or administration. Concordance acts as a safeguard against medication errors in a number of ways:

- In a concordant relationship, where medicine-taking is discussed and patients feel able to be open about their medicine-taking behaviour, overprescribing is less likely. This is because prescribers have a more realistic picture of the medicine that patients are actually taking, and are less likely to add a medicine or increase the dose in the mistaken belief that the current amount prescribed is inadequate to produce the required clinical effect. Examples of this include medication to lower blood pressure.
- A thorough, concordant discussion of medicines is more likely to include over-the-counter and complementary remedies, some of which can cause potentially dangerous interactions with prescribed medication such as aspirin and warfarin.
- Informed agreement about medicines, where risks and benefits are understood, reduces the possibility of patients varying their dose in potentially dangerous ways, without the knowledge of their health professional, such as suddenly discontinuing an antiepilepsy drug.
- Patients who understand their own medicines are better placed to identify and prevent dispensing or administration errors. There are a number of examples of this happening, including vigilant parents who have prevented accidental overdosing of their children with insulin in hospital through their own knowledge of what the correct dose should be.

The significance of concordance in improving the safe use of medicines is beginning to be recognised. The National Patient Safety Agency (NPSA) was amongst the first organisations to sign up to and support Ask About Medicines Week. Its major contribution was to fund the production and evaluation of a pocket-sized patient safety card containing key questions to ask about your medicines, to be distributed through the NHS, pharmacy and other outlets during Ask About Medicines Week.

The NPSA's current priority is the establishment of the national incident reporting system. In addition, it is to be hoped that the NPSA will continue to support and champion concordance as an important contributor to the reduction of medication errors and the safer use of medicines.

The enduring core principles of the NHS, to be found in the NHS Plan (Department of Health, 2000), include as number two the aspiration that NHS services should, in addition to being clinically excellent, be designed around the needs of patients, their families and their carers. From this principle flows a whole range of policies, roles and structures intended to prioritise patient experience and increase public involvement in the NHS. There is now a Director of Patient Experience and Public Involvement, and a Commission for Patient and Public Involvement as well as a range of functions at the local level such as Patient Forums and the Patient Advice and Liaison Service (PALS).

For there to be meaningful involvement by patients and the public in the NHS, relationships need to change at three levels:

1. Strategically, patients and the public need to have a say in setting local and national priorities. Examples of this include lay non-executive members on the boards of PCTs, acute trusts and Strategic Health Authorities, and patient group representatives on the External Reference Groups responsible for developing NSFs.
2. Patient and public experience of health services must be routinely captured and understood so that those who design and deliver services on a day-to-day basis can understand how they are experienced by patients and their families ('the patient's end of the telescope'). Examples include Acute Trust and PCT patient surveys and NSF implementation surveys.
3. Patients must have the opportunity to share in decisions about treatment and be partners in their own care. Examples include concordance and the Expert Patient Programme.

Public and patient involvement is useful shorthand for something that is really about a fundamental redrawing of the relationship between individuals and the health service. In this context, the third level may be the most important of the three because, however many questionnaires are filled in, however many 'ordinary people' sit on NHS boards and committees, the transformation will only be complete when every person is listened to with respect by the health professional who treats them. Concordance fits perfectly into this third level of the hierarchy and, perhaps uniquely of the mechanisms mentioned above, offers a real possibility of enabling every individual patient to experience the public and patient involvement agenda personally and benefit from it in a direct way.

In its entirety, increasing patient and public involvement in the NHS is a daunting enterprise. It is easier to fall back on structural solutions – new roles and bodies, both national and local – than fundamentally to change the culture so that the views and wishes of patients are genuinely listened to and respected at every level of the service. Concordance has a valuable part to play because it combines a subtle change in the relationships between individuals and the service, with a specific outcome – agreement about medicines. Concordance is therefore more tangible than an abstract notion like patient empowerment and, if implemented, has the potential to affect directly many more patients than a new structure, such as PALS (Royal Pharmaceutical Society of Great Britain, 1997). This makes concordance an excellent starting point for the third level in the public and patient involvement model described above. Medicines concordance can function as a catalyst, because once patients are partners in relation to their medicines, genuinely informed agreement about other aspects of care is bound to follow.

Research and development (R&D)

The origin of concordance is as a research-led concept. It was by critically examining the literature on the scale and consequences of non-compliance, its causes and solutions, with the help of social scientists, that the idea of concordance emerged. The evidence base on non-compliance is huge but, unsurprisingly, its quality is mixed.

Looking for data on compliance issues in specific patient populations is currently more or less a fruitless exercise – whether this is defined by age, ethnicity or any other demographic variable. This is despite the fact that we are well aware of particular health problems in some of our black and minority ethnic communities and we know that health beliefs are an important influence on medicine-taking (Horne and Weinman, 1999).

The evidence base on interventions which improve compliance is also very thin, particularly given the interest there has been in this subject over many years. Fewer than 20 trials met the rigorous criteria for inclusion in the Cochrane review (Haynes *et al.*, 2002), which concluded that simple provision of information did not increase compliance and that multifaceted interventions were more likely to be effective, although overall the evidence of effectiveness of any particular approach is equivocal. To some extent, however, the few eligible studies identified reflect a relatively recent increased understanding of the most appropriate methodologies to be applied to the topic, and in this regard, research into compliance is no different from much other health services research.

The conclusion from this should be that there is still an urgent need for research into a reliable predictive framework to identify prospectively non-compliance, and to prove the value of concordance in terms of satisfaction, health outcome and cost. This is covered in more detail in Chapter 7. Sadly for us, funding research is not part of the remit of the current Task Force on Medicines Partnership. The Task Force role in R&D is mainly confined to drawing on the existing evidence base to identify strategies for putting concordance into practice, and developing approaches to measure and audit results, the second of these being significantly more difficult than the first.

Pilots and model practice

One of the most challenging objectives for the Task Force over its 2-year programme was the requirement to demonstrate the potential for putting concordance into practice and producing measurable benefits within the NHS. This was exacerbated by the lack of a universally accepted conceptual model of concordance in a 'real-world' practice setting. Given the relatively modest budget it was obvious from the outset that the Task Force was not in a position to fund pilot projects on any significant scale. It was equally clear that, in the absence of a well-defined blueprint of how concordance should operate in practice, a relatively open approach was needed. The aim was therefore to encourage experimentation and distil learning from a variety of different approaches, with a view to discovering what works and being able to make some definitive recommendations by the end of the 2-year period. This dictated a tripartite approach to promoting the practical implementation of concordance:

1. identifying and supporting existing concordance projects, in as wide a variety of settings and sectors as possible
2. facilitating a small number of selected new projects in high-priority areas where there was limited existing activity and where the potential for generalisable learning was perceived to be highest
3. disseminating results and sharing learning within the concordance community and beyond it

To find and make contact with existing concordance projects, the Task Force engaged in an active networking programme, which included a range of articles in the professional and industry press, conference presentations, small meetings and seminars, and visits to individual companies and PCTs that were already active or interested in concordance. The Task Force also put out a formal Call for Projects which defined the criteria for projects to carry the Medicines Partnership brand, and described the benefits which a formal association with the Task Force might offer.

This process has generated a number of useful insights for the Task Force, and has paved the way to a varied and interesting portfolio of projects. The first surprise that emerged from the initial response to the Call for Projects was the widespread and continued misunderstanding attached to the term 'concordance', even among organisations and individuals who might be expected by now to have arrived at a reasonable grasp of the concept. The term 'concordance' is still commonly used as a substitute for compliance or its softer alternative, adherence. In this sense it appears to have taken on the function of the word 'compliance' while at the same time implying that the speaker/writer is *au fait* with the new terminology and, furthermore, recognises that blaming the patient for not taking the medicine is no longer the appropriate response – compliance with a smiling face. This interpretation resulted in the Task Force receiving a large number of submissions for potential projects aimed at helping people take their medicines as the doctor intended, whether through persuasion, patient education or the use of compliance aids.

Another strong feature has been the number of project submissions that would be classed as pure research rather than demonstrating the results of a specific intervention. Most of these seem to be attempting to find out why people are not complying, rather than testing ways to improve compliance through the practical application of concordance. There seems little reason to believe that any of these projects are likely to yield new insights into the underlying causes of non-compliance as none appears to be testing any particularly new or radical hypotheses and few have demonstrated a thorough grasp of what is already known in this area. This seems to point to a problem in defining what can usefully be achieved in local, practical experiments. There is certainly a role for practitioners and non-academics to push back the frontiers of what is known about effective health services, but research and practice development are not interchangeable. A distinction needs to be made between what can legitimately be learned on a small scale in a practical setting – mostly about the feasibility and impact of process change – and what is better explored with larger samples and more rigorous methodologies.

In addition to its primary role in developing new drugs, the pharmaceutical industry has shown itself to be a source of innovation in supporting people taking medicines. A number of companies have designed and implemented initiatives designed to support patients taking specific medicines, for obvious commercial reasons. Two examples are the Roche MAP programme for orlistat (Xenical) and Biogen's work on beta-interferon. The results from some of these programmes in terms of compliance and patient satisfaction look very promising. Industry has learned through practical experience, rather than as a matter of theory or principle, that programmes which seek to encourage medicine-taking in a paternalistic way generally fail. In other words, for most of us, being reminded, however politely and supportively, to take our medicine because it does us good, will have little effect. In contrast, being proactive and available to answer questions, discuss problems and reassure, particularly in the first few weeks after the prescription, would seem, for some conditions and treatments, to be a highly effective strategy. One might reasonably ask why, if such approaches can be shown to satisfy patients, improve outcomes and have a positive cost–benefit, they are not available as an integral part of the NHS.

Conclusion

The Task Force on Medicines Partnership was established not because concordance is an elegant theory, nor because involving patients is the latest NHS orthodoxy, but on the basis of a hypothesis that, in the end, concordance would lead to measurable, cost-effective improvements in patient care and satisfaction. Given the resources that are spent each year developing and prescribing medicines, half of which are not taken as prescribed, the size of the concordance prize is potentially huge. The practical effect of concordance is unknown. It may be an increase in compliance, with more medicines being taken, and consequent health gain. Alternatively, it may mean less medication that is not actually going to be taken by patients prescribed, dispensed and wasted. Or, it may result in fewer, more effective medicines replacing many less effective ones. Whichever one or combination of these turns out to be the case, the acid test for concordance is whether it can be shown to work in practice. Demonstrating this should be the real determinant of the future of concordance.

References

Anonymous (2003). British pharmaceutical conference: new ways of involving patients. *Pharm J* 271: 519–521.

Audit Commission (2001). *Change Here! Managing Change to Improve Local Services*. London: Audit Commission.

Department for Education and Skills (2003). *The National Literacy Strategy*. Available online at www.standards.dfes.gov.uk/literacy (accessed 12/11/2003).

Department of Health (2000). *The NHS Plan*. London: Department of Health.

Department of Health (2001a). *Pharmacy in the Future: Implementing the NHS Plan – A Programme for Pharmacy in the National Health Service*. London: Department of Health.

Department of Health (2001b). *The Expert Patient: a New Approach to Chronic Disease Management for the 21st Century*. London: Department of Health.

Department of Health (2001c). *Medicines and Older People: Implementing Medicines-Related Aspects of the NSF for Older People*. London: Department of Health.

Department of Health (2001d). *An Organisation With A Memory*. London: Department of Health.

Department of Health (2003). *Supplementary Prescribing by Nurses and Pharmacists Within the NHS in England. A Guide for Implementation*. London: Department of Health.

Haynes R B, McDonald H, Garg A X, Montague P (2002). *Interventions for Helping Patients to Follow Prescriptions for Medications*. Oxford: Cochrane Library.

Horne R, Weinman J (1999). Patients' beliefs about prescribed medicines and their role in adherence to treatment in chronic illness. *J Psychosom Res* 47 (6): 555–567.

Marinker M, Shaw J (2003). Not to be taken as directed. *BMJ* 326: 348–349.

Medicines Partnership (2002). *Room for Review. A Guide to Medication Review: The Agenda for Patients, Practitioners and Managers*. London: Medicines Partnership.

Medicines Partnership (2003). *A Question of Choice: Compliance in Medicine Taking*. London: Medicines Partnership.

Raynor D K, Savage I, Knapp P, Henley J (2003). We are the experts: people with asthma talk about their medicine information needs. Patient Education and Counselling (in press).

Royal Pharmaceutical Society of Great Britain (1997). *From Compliance to Concordance*. London: RPSGB.

White C (2003). Doctors fail to grasp concept of concordance. *BMJ* 327: 642.

Index

Note: page numbers in *italics* refer to boxes, figures and tables.